THE
ASTHMA
SELF-CARE
BOOK

THE
ASTHMA
SELF-CARE
BOOK

How to Take Control of Your Asthma

GERI HARRINGTON

HarperPerennial
A Division of HarperCollins*Publishers*

Asthma self-care depends on a broad understanding of the nature of the disease and a specific understanding of which management techniques work for you. It is important to realize that, no matter how knowledgeable you become, you can never know as much as your own physician. An important part of successful self-care includes knowing when to seek professional advice. We hope this book will help you achieve control of your asthma, but it is in no way intended to substitute for your physician's care. Always check with your doctor before implementing any of the information provided herein.

A hardcover edition of this book was published in 1991 by HarperCollins Publishers.

HarperCollins books may be purchased for educational, business, or sales promotional use. For information, please call or write: Special Markets Department, HarperCollins Publishers, Inc., 10 East 53rd Street, New York, NY 10022. Telephone: (212) 207-7528; Fax: (212) 207-7222.

First HarperPerennial edition published 1992.

Designed by Alma Orenstein

The Library of Congress has catalogued the hardcover edition as follows:

Harrington, Geri.
    Asthma self-care book: how to take control of your asthma/Geri Harrington.—1st ed.
      p. cm.
    Includes index.
    ISBN 0-06-016584-7:
    1. Asthma—Popular works. 2. Self-care, Health—Popular works.
    I. Title.
    RC591.H37   1991
    616.2'38—dc20   90-55538

ISBN 0-06-092270-2 (pbk.)

92 93 94 95 96 MB 10 9 8 7 6 5 4 3 2 1

To Margaret Haggerty, R.N., M.S.N.

Contents

Foreword

We are on the brink of a new age—the information age—and, in medicine, this means changes in the management of disease that will affect doctors and patients alike. Doctors will no longer be taught to memorize masses of data; instead they will learn how to retrieve the information they need quickly, easily, and accurately from the computer. More and more medical schools will, as Johns Hopkins is already doing, choose aspiring physicians on the basis not just of test scores but also of the degree to which they are temperamentally and emotionally suited to practice their chosen profession.

Patients will have to adjust to doctors who expect them to take responsibility for their own care. In many instances, as with asthma for example, it will no longer be acceptable for a patient to say, "Doctor, make me well." Such a request is likely to be met with the response, "No—you are going to make yourself well—with my help."

The old-fashioned passive dependence on the physician will apply only to such illnesses as pneumonia, where there is little the patient can do except follow instructions, confident that appropriate medical care is forthcoming. But with a chronic disease such

as asthma the patient is an important part of the team and must
pull his or her own weight.

If you wish to be well, give thought to your illness, not pas-
sively but in a spirit of cooperation. With your doctor's help,
you—and your family—can learn to understand the nature of
your disease, recognize the significance of your symptoms, and
manage them. You need not be afraid to ask your doctor questions, but once you understand the reasons for and the nature of
your treatment, bend every effort to complying with them.

In the last fifteen years we have taken giant steps toward
understanding the underlying causes of asthma—although we still
do not fully understand it—and more and more emphasis is being
put on prevention. Initially, of course, you will be more anxious
to learn how to control bronchospasm and wheezing and the
other unpleasant aspects of an asthma attack, but you will soon
come to appreciate the feeling of control you have over the disease when you find you can more and more frequently anticipate
incidents and stop them from occurring in the first place.

This knowledge, concerning the prevention and cure of the
factors that cause asthma, is just as important as the treatment of
asthma itself. Failure to recognize the important contemporary
causes of asthma can result in peristent and progressive asthmatic
conditions leading to unnecessary and even dangerous dependence on drug therapy. The major causes of asthma, other than
the usual allergies, are well known and can be effectively treated.
These include viral infections of the bronchial tree, exposure to
noxious gases and chemicals, infection of the sinuses, and sensitivity to chemicals in industry. The best treatment for asthma
caused by exposure to chemicals in the workplace is control of the
environment or total avoidance of the offending problem. In order
to achieve this, there should be complete and truthful communication between the patient and the physician.

To work intelligently with your physician, you must have a
background of knowledge to call on. Doctors have the knowledge
you need but do not always have the time or the ability to trans-
late it into terms that are accessible to the patient, and so you may
often leave the doctor's office without a clear idea of what you

need to know to take care of your asthma yourself.

Asthma Self-Care, written by Geri Harrington, who has asthma but who is also a medical writer, provides a hands-on point of view not generally found in books on this subject. It provides the full spectrum of the knowledge you need, in language you can understand, so that you can enjoy a happier, healthier, fuller life. With the help of this book you can, through self-care, look forward to achieving a measure of control over your asthma that you may never have thought possible. I wish you every success.

Sreedhar Nair, M.D.

Chief, Section of Pulmonary and Critical
    Care, Norwalk Hospital, Norwalk,
    Connecticut
Clinical Professor, Yale University
    School of Medicine
President, National Emphysema
    Foundation

Preface

I decided to write this book when I was about to be discharged from the hospital after a near brush with death from an attack of status asthmaticus. My doctor sternly admonished me, "I don't want to see you land in the hospital in this condition again," and I knew what he meant. He was telling me that my experience had been due entirely to not calling for help quickly enough—and that it had been completely unnecessary.

My only health problem up to then had been seasonal hay fever, plus a few mild allergies to cats and dust. Asthma was a minor inconvenience that occurred intermittently, and in the beginning my doctor prescribed a Ventolin inhaler that took care of it. Gradually, though I was unaware of the pattern, I began to get bronchitis every November (at the end of the worst of the hay fever), and he added Theo-Dur tablets to my medication regimen.

I had never taken my occasional breathing problems seriously. It didn't occur to me that I could have an attack that could get out of control or that anyone could die from asthma. Usually when I began to have trouble breathing, I walked through it by going for a stroll in the woods. That's what I had done this time, but the walk had only made it worse, and I came home even more uncomfortable, with increasing anxiety. I tried to relax, turning on the radio while I made something to eat. The radio said a smoke inversion from forest fires down south was blanketing my area, and "anyone with respiratory problems is advised to stay indoors." So I knew then why the walk hadn't helped and assumed being indoors, taking it easy, and using the medication would take care of matters.

By the time I realized I actually couldn't take another breath, my son had called the ambulance. I blacked out as it came down the driveway.

Although I write about medical subjects and have a library of basic medical reference books, I was almost totally ignorant about asthma. When I got out of the hospital, I joined a pulmonary rehabilitation group, started to attend breathing clubs at the American Lung Association and Norwalk Hospital, and began to talk to doctors and respiratory rehabilitation nurse/therapists. But most of all, I talked to other people with asthma.

What I learned is that the majority of asthmatics don't know a lot about asthma either. But since asthma is a chronic disease, most of the time they still have to take care of themselves. They see a doctor only when they decide they need to, and—as I almost demonstrated—unless you understand what asthma is all about, it's possible for that decision to come too late.

So I have written this book for everyone who has asthma, or who has family or friends with asthma. I hope you all will discover in these pages that asthma is truly reversible and generally controllable, and that almost no one need die of it or even let it interfere with a normal, active, and basically healthy life.

Acknowledgments

This book could not have been written without the help of the many busy and dedicated physicians, scientists, nurse/therapists, and pharmacists who freely took the time to answer my innumerable questions and during lengthy interviews and follow-up phone consults generously gave me the benefit of their knowledge and expertise.

Among them, I would especially like to thank the following: Robert D. Ballard, M.D., staff physician, Department of Medicine, National Jewish Center for Immunology and Respiratory Medicine, Denver, Colorado; Maryanne Bartoszek, M.D.; Paul Beres, M.D.; Margaret Haggerty, R.N., M.S.N.; Joel Kabak, M.D.; Michael A. Kaliner, M.D., National Institute of Allergic and Infectious Diseases, Bethesda, Maryland; Gary L. Larsen, M.D., pediatric pulmonology, National Jewish Center for Immunology and Respiratory Medicine; Donald M. Mecca, R. Ph.; Henry Milgrom, M.D., staff physician, Department of Pediatrics, National Jewish Center for Immunology and Respiratory Medicine; Bruce D. Miller, M.D., pediatric psychiatry, National Jewish Center for Immunology and Respiratory Medicine; Harold S. Nelson, M.D., staff physician, Department of Medicine, National Jewish Center for Immunology

and Respiratory Medicine; Mark W. Osowski, R. Ph.; Sidney
Parker, Ph.D., Chief, Prevention and Research Training Program,
Division of Lung Diseases, National Heart, Lung, and Blood Institute, Bethesda, Maryland; Gordon Raphael, M.D., National Institute
of Allergic and Infectious Diseases; Manuel Sanguily, M.D.; Michael Sly, M.D., Children's Hospital, Washington, D.C.; Jeanne
(Dee-Dee) C. Vallez, R.N., M.S., A.N.P., clinical specialist/nurse
educator, National Jewish Center for Immunology and Respiratory Medicine; and Eva Wilson, R.R.T.

In addition, I would like to thank Robert Fuentes, Pharm. D.,
Glaxo, Inc. (U.S.), and Dan Quinn, B. Sc., Glaxo, Canada, for the
time they took to talk with me and the wealth of material they sent.

Special mention is also due the entire network of the American Lung Association. I was overwhelmed by the warm response
to the request for information I sent to each state chapter, and the
generous help that was forthcoming, state by state around the
country.

And not least of all, I would like to thank the many asthma
patients I met who did not hesitate to share their experiences with
me, and who provided insight into their needs, their medical
relationships, and what information they would find useful. I hope
in reading this book, they will feel I listened well.

Part One

Getting Started with Self-Care

1

Introduction to Asthma and Self-Care

What Is Asthma?

Asthma is a chronic disease that presently affects an estimated ten to fifteen million Americans of all ages. Incidence of asthma is increasing, and although widespread air pollution is thought to be a factor, the cause of this increase is not really known. Fortunately, compared with other chronic diseases, asthma has a number of characteristics in its favor. Dr. Harold S. Nelson, senior staff physician at National Jewish Center for Immunology and Respiratory Medicine in Denver, speaks from considerable experience when he says, "Asthma is reversible and can be controlled."

Another favorable aspect of the disease is that a person with asthma can be healthy and normal when not experiencing symptoms. "With good medical treatment and conscientious self-care most asthmatics can lead normal lives," assures Dr. Nelson. In the absence of active symptoms even a physical examination may not reveal any signs of asthma; lungs and airways may appear completely normal. Sophisticated tests sometimes reveal physiological changes in the lungs of asthmatics, but the effect on the body of such changes is not known, and they are not invariably present.

There is no cure for asthma as yet, but considerable progress has been made in recent years in diagnosis and treatment, and ongoing research promises the possibility of even better management in the near future. An important advance in treatment was made when the focus of research changed from decreasing the severity of the symptoms to preventing them from occurring. In the past a person with asthma was treated and given medication only when wheezing and shortness of breath occurred; today medications are prescribed on a maintenance schedule that aims at keeping the patient free of these symptoms. Since an important part of prevention is not only drugs but also diet and exercise, this new approach benefits the whole body, and asthmatics who faithfully follow this enlightened regimen may easily end up healthier than many of their nonasthmatic counterparts.

What Causes Asthma?

We still do not know the underlying causes of asthma, but we are beginning to understand what sets off symptoms and the physiological processes that take place when the symptoms occur.

We call the substance or activity that sets off asthma symptoms a "trigger," and we know that although some things are more liable to cause trouble than others, triggers can be almost anything. Years ago it was thought that all asthma was due to allergens, but that turned out to be only part of the story. We now know there are two basic types of asthma: extrinsic—caused by allergy triggers, such as pollen and pets—and intrinsic—caused by nonallergic triggers, such as an inflammation, a sinus infection, a cold, stress, or exercise. What constitutes a trigger varies from person to person, even within a family.

According to Dr. Michael A. Kaliner of the National Institute of Allergic and Infectious Diseases, about 90 percent of children's asthma is extrinsic, whereas only 50 percent of adults fall into this category. It is possible, however, to have both kinds of asthma simultaneously. (See Chapter 12, "Recognizing and Dealing with Asthma Triggers.")

Because stress tends to exacerbate asthma, it used to be thought that perhaps asthma was a psychosomatic disease. It is now understood that stress is a trigger that can cause asthma symptoms or make them worse, but that it will not give someone asthma or cause symptoms in anyone who does not already have the disease. A nonasthmatic will never get an asthma attack, no matter how upset or stressed he or she becomes.

What Happens When You Get an Attack?

The characteristic symptoms of asthma—shortness of breath, a tight feeling in the chest, wheezing, and difficulty breathing—are due partly to constriction of the muscles wrapped around the bronchial tubes (bronchospasm). In addition, the lining of the bronchial tubes (mucosa) swells and becomes inflamed, and an increase of thick, sticky mucus is produced. These three changes in the bronchial tubes narrow them so that there is less space for air to get through. The effort to force air through this narrowed space may cause the wheezing sound associated with asthma. If, however, the attack is severe enough so that no air gets through, there is no wheezing.

Coughing may occur in an effort to bring up the sticky mucus that is clogging the airways; if it is nonproductive, it may increase the constriction.

When air cannot easily get in or out, more air than usual (some air is always unexpelled) inevitably becomes trapped in the lungs, leaving less room for fresh, oxygenated air to get in. There is normally less resistance when breathing in than when breathing out, and during an asthmatic attack, although you may feel you are trying to breathe air in, breathing air out is what has really become critical.

Long before you reach this point, you will probably have used your inhaler, reversed the bronchospasm by relaxing the bronchial muscles, and restored normal breathing. If, however, there is much inflammation and you are not taking medication to reduce it, you may have a subsequent attack (the pulmonary late-phase response or late-phase reaction) because of the inflammation. With proper management this need not happen.

The Pulmonary Late-Phase Response

An asthma episode usually happens immediately or very shortly (fifteen to thirty minutes) after exposure to a trigger. Once the symptoms are brought under control and normal breathing has been attained, most asthmatics would expect that to be the end of it. What can sometimes happen, though, is that while the bronchospasm may have been reversed, the airways are left with a hidden, inflammatory condition that lasts much longer. In this case, several hours or even days later, a second episode may occur (the late-phase response) that is actually a continuation of the original one, although it may not be recognized as such.

This kind of asthmatic episode is not yet clearly understood, but we do know some things about it. You may wonder how it differs from any other kind of episode, and why you can't ignore what it is called and simply control it as you would any ordinary attack. The reason is that it is different in ways that are necessary for you to understand.

Dr. Gary L. Larsen, pediatric pulmonologist at the National Jewish Center for Immunology and Respiratory Medicine, explains why it is difficult to recognize late-phase attacks but important to do so. "In their bare symptoms a pulmonary late-phase response and an immediate asthmatic reaction are much alike. The patient experiences chest tightness, dyspnea [difficulty in breathing], and wheezing, although the airway obstruction can be so severe that audible wheezing is absent. The most obvious differences lie in their time of onset and duration. . . . The immediate reaction resolves within an hour or two, even if no medication is given; the late-phase response may last for several hours, and sometimes for days." The late-phase response is also always very troublesome and resembles chronic, severe asthma. Aside from the severity of the attack, the clue you may have that you are experiencing late-phase response asthma is that bronchodilators (anticholinergic, sympathomimetic, or theophylline drugs), which normally work, are not as effective as usual. Fortunately, two drugs you may have on hand, steroids and cromolyn sodium (Intal), are very effective in blocking late-response asthma.

Late-phase response is not uncommon. Dr. Larsen says that "several studies of the incidence of late responses in atopic patients [showed] a rate of 50 percent."

The Peak-Flow Meter

It's all very well to understand what happens when you get an attack, but it is obviously better not to get one at all. Having a peak-flow meter on hand is an easy way to keep track of how you are doing.

This simple, hand-held device measures your peak expiratory flow rate—in other words, how much air you can blow out of your lungs in one second. It is easy for anyone to use, even a child; all you do is take a deep breath while holding it in front of your mouth, then blow out as hard and as fast as you can. The blowing out should be very quick; if you keep on blowing, you are wasting your time, because only the first hard, fast breath counts. This is easy to see when you use it: the marker is moved by your first burst of breath and does not continue to move if you continue breathing. Be sure to move the marker back to zero after you have read it. If you don't, your next reading may amaze you by edging up higher than your best baseline!

My rehab respiratory therapist always used a peak-flow meter at the beginning and end of each session and strongly urged me to buy one, but I had never quite gotten around to it. When I started doing research for this book, Dr. Nelson told me, "A peak-flow meter is absolutely invaluable. Everyone with asthma should have one." He also felt it was important to learn how to use it properly. He showed me a number of studies and charts, demonstrating how charting an asthmatic's daily peak flow would signal deteriorating breathing or, conversely, show that the person had been stabilized and was doing well.

To read a peak-flow meter, look at where the marker is; a number tells you what your peak-flow rate was. Again, always move the marker back to zero. Repeat the hard, fast breath three times—there shouldn't be much difference if you are doing it right—and count the highest reading. There are different designs of peak-flow meters, but they all work the same way to provide an objective evaluation of how well or poorly you are breathing.

Since you are comparing yourself to yourself, it is helpful if at some point you do it when you are feeling quite well so that you get a baseline reading. Then any deviation from that, especially a reading that drops more than 20 percent, warns you that something is amiss and should be brought to your doctor's attention.

Always take your reading before medicating or using a bronchodilator or inhaler. And always do it at the same time, preferably as soon as you get up in the morning. Depending on the severity of your asthma, your doctor may want you to use the meter twice a day (be sure the evening reading is also done before taking any medication) and to write the results in a log. Once you are stabilized, he or she may be satisfied with less frequent readings.

Another use for this handy little device is monitoring medication results. If you think your medication is not as effective as the doctor expected, it's easy enough to check, using your baseline as a guide. On the other hand, if you feel so much better that you think perhaps you can reduce your dosage, a few days' readings might confirm your opinion (but don't change your regimen without discussing it with your doctor).

A peak-flow meter is also useful when you think you are getting a cold or a "bug." It will quickly indicate a lower-than-normal reading if you are coming down with something and alert you to the desirability of calling the doctor.

Another use for the meter is to try to develop an awareness

of your health. Generally, subjective judgments as to whether your asthma is bothering you are not very accurate. Surprisingly, it works both ways; you may feel fine and actually be breathing poorly, or you may feel breathless and measure up to your baseline. Sometimes using the peak-flow meter for a while may help you develop a more accurate feel of the state of your breathing. If you're never sure you're evaluating yourself correctly, don't worry about it; the nice thing is that with a peak-flow meter handy you don't have to.

There is no question in my mind that if I had been using a peak-flow meter regularly, or even just had one in the house to turn to when I started to feel uncomfortable, I would never have found myself being intubated in an ambulance on Route 7 in the middle of a November night. Instead, at worst, I could have realized what was happening in time to drive myself to the emergency room, gotten treatment, and been back in my own bed before dawn.

Aside from all its practical uses, the feeling of security that comes with having a peak-flow meter on hand is worth a lot to people who have a disease that tends to create anxiety. It's comparatively inexpensive, but check around before you buy one. Pharmacies differ in what they charge, and if you belong to a respiratory rehab center, they usually have them available for less than the drugstore price.

Why Do Asthma Symptoms Occur?

We do not know what causes asthma, but we do know that asthma triggers cause asthma symptoms. We also know how.

Asthma is often described as "an overactive immune system." The immune system's function is to protect the body against invaders that are perceived as harmful; anything that appears to threaten the health of the body activates the immune system, which rushes to defend it by attacking the invaders. When you have asthma, your immune system overreacts—perceives harmless things as threats—and this perception triggers an inappropriate reaction from the immune system's defense mechanisms, causing the symptoms.

The most noticeable symptom, bronchospasm, is really the end result of a chemical process that may have begun some time before you are aware of it.

Let's take a simple example. Say you have extrinsic (allergic) asthma, and one of your potential allergens is ragweed. Every day you pass a field where ragweed grows. One day it is in flower, and the air is full of ragweed pollen. If this is your first encounter, nothing may happen. After subsequent exposure, however, you "become allergic" to ragweed pollen (but only if ragweed is an allergen for you; it isn't for everyone).

When you develop the allergy, ragweed pollen is identified by your immune system as a harmful foreign substance. The soldiers of your immune system army are white blood cells. There are many kinds; the kind we are interested in at the moment produces antibodies (specialized proteins called immunoglobulins), which they release into the blood. What is special about antibodies is that they are programmed to attack only one allergen, in this case ragweed pollen. (A different antibody is produced for each allergen, and it will not attack any other antigen, or substance capable of inducing an immune response.)

The type of antibody produced against ragweed pollen is called immunoglobulin E, or IgE (there are four other kinds), and it attaches its Y-shaped molecules around the outside of a special kind of cell called a mast cell (which is usually described, at that point, as looking like a pincushion full of pins). Mast cells are found inside the nose and throughout the tracheobronchial tree, which includes the airways. When the ragweed pollen is inhaled, it attaches to the IgE antibodies that are sticking out from the mast cell, causing the mast cell to release strong chemicals called mediators into the tissues lining the nose and airway, damaging them and causing an allergic reaction. Among these mediators is histamine—which explains why one type of drug for countering allergic reactions is called an antihistamine.

The release of histamine can affect a number of areas in the body, depending on where the mast cells are located. If you have asthma, and if histamine is released by mast cells in the airways, it can cause bronchospasm. In addition, as we have noted, other mast cells in the tracheobronchial tree contain many other mediators. Some specifically cause the contraction of airway muscles, increased mucus production, or an increase in white blood cells that produce inflammation—all reactions that are, or are directly related to, the key symptoms of an asthma attack.

In developing drugs to help manage or prevent asthma symptoms, it is necessary to go a step further because the autonomic nervous system (which, among its functions, controls the smooth muscles of the airways as well as the mucus production mechanism) also operates through the chemicals called mediators. In this instance, the mediators act like switches, turning muscle contractions on or off according to the receptors they come in contact with. For example, adrenergic beta-receptors not only relax bronchial muscles but also inhibit the adrenergic alpha-receptors and cholinergic receptors that would otherwise stimulate muscle contraction.

An instance of the practical application of this process for the manufacturer is the development of a drug that blocks the action of acetylcholine, which is the cholinergic mediator. Atrovent (ipratropium bromide) is an example of this type of drug. Drugs with which you may be even more familiar, such as albuterol, terbutaline, and isoproterenol, are beta-stimulators. (See also Chapters 4–9 and 21, which describe specific drugs in detail.)

What Has All This to Do with Self-Care?

Your doctor knows the physiological manifestations of asthma and what the various drugs can do and plans your individual regime of drug medication accordingly. For the purposes of self-care, it helps if you have a working knowledge of how asthma happens and the state of the art in treating it.

Since the first step in bringing asthma under control is the use of medication, it is important to know something about the characteristics of the specific drugs you are taking and understand what to expect from them. When you know that a certain drug (such as albuterol) will bring instant relief from bronchospasm, while another (cromolyn sodium) is ineffectual for that purpose but will help prevent bronchospasm if taken regularly, you will be able to follow your doctor's instructions more intelligently.

What Does Self-Care Involve?

Self-care means just what it says—taking care of yourself. There is a limit to how much doctors or therapists can help you because most of the time they will not be with you. On the other hand, since asthma is a chronic disease, it is a constant companion. Thus an asthmatic who wishes to live a quality life must learn as much as possible about the disease, follow the doctor's instructions, evaluate how well they are working, and know when to seek professional help.

Today more people are becoming aware that they must assume responsibility for their own health. They make an effort to learn about nutrition, to get enough and the right kind of exercise, to minimize stress, which lowers the immune system, and, in general, to lead a "healthy" life.

An asthmatic must do all that and more; he or she must also learn about asthma and how to deal with it. This is not difficult; in fact, it can be very interesting, especially when you realize that you yourself, under your doctor's guidance, can prevent or alleviate attacks by applying what we now know, and even possibly save your own life by realizing when you need more help than you yourself can provide. The best thing about taking charge of your asthma is that doing so will make it possible for you to lead a happier, healthier, more productive life than you ever thought you could.

The purpose of this book is to show you how.

2

What to Do If You Think
You Have Asthma

Asthma often goes undiagnosed; it is estimated that thousands of people have asthma and neither they nor even their doctors are aware of it. There are many reasons: asthma varies with each individual; it is not usually constant; misconceptions abound about the nature of the disease; and its symptoms can sometimes be mistaken for those of other illnesses.

First, if you find yourself getting unusually short of breath, asthma isn't likely to be the first disease that pops into your mind. Many people experiencing shortness of breath think immediately of heart disease. Or if your chest feels tight and you're coughing up mucus, you may decide it's a cold or, if you feel really sick, bronchitis. Since asthma symptoms go away and leave you feeling fine, a brief period of not feeling well will probably not send you to the doctor, and you will forget about them until the next time they occur.

If your child is sick, you are likely to check with the pediatrician whenever an illness seems out of the ordinary. If you're an adult, you can usually evaluate how sick you feel, and if your illness seems unusual or very uncomfortable, you may give the doctor a call to tell him or her about it. Most of the time an adult does not pay attention to asthma until it starts to be a noticeable bother. And with extrinsic asthma, if your symptoms are seasonal, you may dismiss the problem as hay fever.

Unlike the case with many other chronic illnesses, it is not necessarily harmful if asthma is not diagnosed in its very early stages. It is not inevitable that it will get worse; with luck it may stay mild or appear to go away and not recur for years. If, however, your symptoms become more frequent and more uncomfortable, or if you have a real attack, no matter how mild, you should see a doctor.

The Primary Care Physician

If you already have a family doctor, start with him or her. It is always better not to try to self-diagnose your condition. You may guess wrong, and if you bypass your family doctor and go to a specialist, you may waste your time and money if your diagnosis is incorrect and your illness does not fall under that specialty.

A family doctor may be a general practitioner, a doctor specializing in family practice, or an internist. Many internists are now routinely used as "family doctors" by people who do not always realize that internists are specialists in internal medicine. (They are not to be confused with interns, who are graduate medical students completing their training by residing and serving in a hospital.)

Whatever your family doctor is, he—or she—is your primary care physician, and if you have been his patient for any length of time, he is the person who knows your medical history and has a fairly good idea of your general physical condition.

If he is an internist, determine whether he has a subspecialty; more and more internists do. (You can find out by looking him up in the telephone directory yellow pages, where it may be listed after his name.) It's a good idea to know what your internist's subspecialty is. In the beginning it may not make much difference because asthma is a very common disease, and many doctors who are not pulmonary specialists can do an excellent job of managing it. As long as he doesn't limit his practice to his subspecialty, he still can be your primary care physician.

When you consult a family practitioner or an internist without an active subspecialty, keep in mind that his strength is that he is a generalist, with a knowledge of the whole broad field of medicine. The advantage he will have over other specialists is that he has a wider viewpoint and can consider your problem in terms of the whole body. Patients often complain that doctors think of them as organs rather than as human beings. In other words, the focus is on the heart, kidney, gallbladder or whatever organ is giving trouble. Your primary care physician is less liable to do that.

Because of his broader viewpoint, your primary care physician should have another important skill: he should be a good diagnostician. Since he is the one who may recommend that you see a specialist, which specialist you see will depend largely on his diagnosis.

The Pediatrician

If you have a young child, you probably have a pediatrician as the child's primary care physician. The pediatrician's role is the same as that described above for the primary care physician. Referrals to allergists and other specialists would also occur in the same way, except that a pediatrician might know of allergists who specialize in children, and who may be better able to interpret treatments for asthma in terms of the special requirements of children.

The Pulmonary Specialist

The primary care physician can manage many cases of asthma and, because it is a fairly common disease, has often had considerable experience with it. But advances in medicine and medical technology are taking place so rapidly that it is impossible for one person to keep completely current in every area.

Since a pulmonary specialist concentrates on respiratory and immunological problems, he, or she, can keep up with the latest technology, the newest tests, the most recently developed medications, as they relate to asthma; by narrowing his focus, he is able to increase the depth of his knowledge in his chosen field. He will not replace your primary care physician but he will add another dimension to your general care.

Do not be surprised if the pulmonary specialist suggests you see an allergist. It doesn't mean he will no longer treat your asthma; it may just be that he thinks you have extrinsic asthma, and your actual allergies can best be treated by an allergist. He will work very closely with the allergist, and your care will be coordinated between them.

The Allergist

An allergist may be an internist or pediatrician who has taken additional training, usually two years, in order to qualify as a specialist in allergy and immunology. Because of the requirement for prior training (as internist or pediatrician), some experts suggest that a patient with severe asthma is best served by having an allergist as the primary care physician. In that case, if you encountered other health problems, such as heart disease, you would presumably be referred to specialists in those areas when appropriate.

Choosing a Doctor

The doctor-patient relationship is a combination of the personal and the impersonal. Doctors are too busy to be closely involved with their patients' lives and "always be there" for them. On the other hand, you have to depend on the doctor when you are sick, which is not a time when you are feeling confident, optimistic, and able to cope. A doctor has to have empathy and understanding and the ability to reassure you. You have to be able to trust him, or her, and feel he cares about your concerns and, possibly, anxieties. In addition, you have to like the doctor and feel he likes you.

If you do not have a good relationship with a doctor or do not feel comfortable with him or the way he works with you, do not hesitate to change doctors. And of course, if you cannot freely discuss his treatment, ask questions, and get clear explanations and instructions, you will not be able to take care of your asthma the way you should. (See also Chapter 10, "How to Work with Your Doctor.")

The Pulmonary Rehabilitation Therapist

A pulmonary rehabilitation team consists of a pulmonary nurse specialist who coordinates the program, a respiratory therapist who helps administer the program, and your doctor. When you join the team (to take part in the pulmonary rehab program), you are on your way to successful self-care. Other professionals, such as a psychiatric nurse clinician, physical and occupational therapists, and a dietitian or nutritionist, are available if needed, but they are not part of the core team that works with you all the time.

The goal of pulmonary rehabilitation is to help you, through education, support, exercise, stress reduction, and other techniques, to manage your asthma so that you can be the best you can be. And the person who works with you toward this goal is a pulmonary rehabilitation therapist, who is a nurse or a respiratory therapist specially trained in pulmonary rehabilitation techniques.

Unlike the treatment doctors usually provide, the tools of pulmonary rehab specialists are not drugs (although they are knowledgeable about them and will help you work with them) but methods that go beyond drugs to help you and your body achieve your maximum level of wellness. They teach you what asthma is, how it reacts under various circumstances, and ways (including knowledgeable use of the drugs your doctor has prescribed) to take an active, rather than a passive, role in managing it.

If you think of drugs—as so many asthmatics do—as necessary but still a kind of crutch, pulmonary rehab will help you to realize that drugs are simply tools to control the symptoms, and using them when you need them is merely sensible, like using a hammer or a screwdriver when it is called for. Best of all, pulmonary rehab helps you get in better physical condition and may make possible activities you thought you could never do again and restore your feeling of independence.

Your own attitude toward helping yourself has everything to do with making pulmonary rehab work. You need to take a truly active role in your own health and be willing to acquire the knowledge you need, apply it on a daily basis, and practice new good habits as you discard old bad habits. Looking at rehab from a cost/benefit viewpoint, there is no question that the cost of the work you will need to do is worth the benefit of improved health and getting back control of your life.

Surprisingly enough, not one of the books on asthma that I have seen to date (granted I may have missed one) lists pulmonary or respiratory therapy in the index. This book does and goes one step better: in Appendix 5 you will find a state-by-state list of pulmonary rehab centers.

Part Two

What the Doctor Can Do

3

The Role of the Physician

You cannot manage asthma without the help of a physician. First of all, asthma must be diagnosed. The human body is capable of a great many symptoms, and only a trained diagnostician can sort them out, discern the pattern, and, with the help of a personal and family medical history, tests, and other information, determine what is causing them. Asthma is characterized by difficulty in breathing and by wheezing. But those symptoms can be due to a number of different diseases; only a physician can tell which one you have.

Once asthma is diagnosed, it can be treated. Although you should be able, with your doctor's help, to manage your own asthma, no matter how knowledgeable you may become you cannot know as much as a trained physician. He or she has access to the latest literature describing ongoing studies throughout the world, attends meetings and seminars where he can compare notes with fellow physicians, is kept up-to-date by pharmaceutical manufacturers on the newest medications, and through medical

21

journals, benefits from the experiences and theories of other physicians in his field. In addition, he has had years of daily, hands-on experience with his own patients and is free to consult with other doctors when he has a question. He knows firsthand, from his own observation, things you could never learn from books. And ideally, he knows a great deal about how the human body works and how asthma fits into the overall picture.

This may not seem to leave much for you to do in the way of self-care, but—as we will see in Part Three—your role is also essential.

Asthma medication plays a key role in the treatment of asthma. Your physician will determine a medication regimen that works for you and will educate you in the application of it. But it is hard to keep in mind everything a doctor tells you in an office visit—even if you take notes—and there are always questions once you have left the office. So a good part of this book is given over to a detailed discussion of most of the medications in use at this time, and what you need to know about them so as to follow your doctor's instructions and use them intelligently.

4

The Role of
Asthma Medications

Many people don't like the idea of taking medication and tend to resist it; the more we become aware of our bodies and want an active role in our health and well-being, the more we tend to feel that there must be a better way than filling ourselves with unfamiliar chemicals. When, in addition, we learn that they have possibly unpleasant or even harmful side effects, it only confirms our first impression that they really aren't good for us, and that we should be able to obtain the same results by living in a healthier way.

Historically, however, the use of drugs to cure disease is not new; man has always looked for remedies to ingest or rub on himself to cure his ailments. Thousands of years ago a Chinese physician became convinced that somewhere in nature there existed an antidote for every illness. He spent a lifetime in the meadows and mountains of China, collecting plant specimens and bringing them back to his village to see whether he could discover what they were good for. Much of the time, in the tradition of medical researchers throughout history, he experimented on himself, and he wrote down the results in notebooks that became the basis of Chinese medicine.

Chinese herbal medicine is still practiced today, and many homeopathic remedies are based on similar theories. Explorers and anthropologists in the remotest areas of the world have found primitive peoples practicing medicine based on natural plant materials, and the indigenous peoples of both North and South America taught colonists effective, "natural" ways of coping with their diseases.

In a way we have come full circle, because modern medications owe much to natural origins. Quinine, digitalis, ergot, and curare, to name just a few, were all known to native peoples and are now, in one form or other, routinely listed among our pharmaceuticals. And even where that is not the case, some of of our medicines are derivatives of substances produced by the body itself, such as insulin, cortisone, and thyroid medications.

What many of the latter have in common is that they seek to fill a need that the body is no longer able to. Insulin injections, to take the most familiar example, help the diabetic whose own production of insulin is insufficient. And asthma medications likewise, though in a different way, function by replicating a chemical process the body is no longer controlling properly. Although you will not be determining or prescribing your own asthma medications, you will be able to follow the doctor's instructions more intelligently if you have some understanding of why he or she has chosen certain drugs for you and what they are expected to do. And you will be better equipped to help the physician determine whether they are working.

The Function of Asthma Medications

To understand the function of asthma medications, you need to know something about the physiological reactions in the body that cause asthma symptoms, such as bronchospasm. With asthma the immune system, which normally protects the body against harmful invaders such as certain bacteria, is overactive and protective to the point of creating a problem where none would otherwise exist. The simplest example is what happens with extrinsic, or allergic, asthma.

As explained in Chapter 1, the first time you breathe in an ordinarily harmless substance, such as pollen or cat dander, that you happen to have become allergic to, it triggers a defense mechanism which creates a welcoming committee, called receptors, on certain cells (mast cells); any further contact with the allergen causes the cells to release chemicals, such as histamine, that through a complicated system of enzymes and other substances produce the physiological symptoms of asthma: bronchospasm, mucus formation, swelling of the airway tissues, and coughing. Although the action of mast cells is incompletely understood, that is approximately the sequence of what is thought to happen, and thus some preventive-action drugs, such as Atrovent, are designed to act as mast-cell stabilizers.

Among the substances the body manufactures are certain "pairs" that act in opposite ways; one, for example, constricts the bronchial tubes while another acts to relax and keep them open. Unfortunately, asthma allergic reactions lean toward the former, so one set of asthma medications is designed to prevent or reverse the bronchospasm, thus opening the airways.

It is thought that the chemical in the body most responsible for controlling the release of (among other things) bronchoconstricting substances like histamine is one called cyclic AMP (cAMP, for short), and that a deficiency of cAMP causes asthma and allergic reactions. One group of medications, known as beta-adrenergic or sympathomimetic agents, is designed specifically to stimulate the production of cAMP, so that when you use, for instance, an albuterol inhaler (Ventolin, Proventil), the effect is to open the airways and bring you immediate relief. Medications that counteract bronchospasm are generally referred to as bronchodilators (see box), and they act like Adrenalin but are more practical for individual use because they can be inhaled or taken in tablet form, whereas Adrenalin can be administered only by injection.

Another group of drugs is designed to achieve the same effect

---
Bronchodilators

There are three types of bronchodilators:

1. sympathomimetic (Adrenalin-like or adrenergic, such as Ventolin and Proventil)
2. anticholinergic (a calcium-blocker and mast-cell stabilizer, such as Atrovent)
3. theophylline (such as Theo-Dur and Slo-Bid)

As we will see when we talk about the drugs in more detail, they differ somewhat in their action, the forms in which they are available, and their side effects.

---

but through a different action of the body. Histamine, for example, cannot be released (and cause bronchospasm) unless there is sufficient calcium present in the cell membranes. While calcium in other instances is a beneficial substance, one of its functions— to aid muscle contraction—is not what we want in this particular context, so preventing calcium access to the cell membranes is desirable. Chemists have developed a group of drugs that do just that. Cromolyn sodium drugs are part of this group and seem, in addition to their effect on calcium, to make the airways less reactive.

Corticosteroids, on the other hand, act in still a third way in an asthma situation. A natural and essential product of the human body, steroids play a very complicated role, but from the standpoint of someone with asthma their two most valuable characteristics at present lie in their ability to prevent inflammation and, during an active episode, to increase the effectiveness of other drugs. When nothing else seems to work, steroids come to the rescue.

Theophylline, which in the United States is commonly the drug of choice, works in yet another way, but the mechanism is not yet completely understood. We know it works, and we think its action is related to the production of cAMP, but we are not sure exactly how.

Trying to manage asthma symptoms without drugs is not recommended; it is extremely difficult at best and in most cases impossible. Once you are symptom-free, your doctor will show you how and how far to cut back, but you are still liable to get into trouble when you encounter an asthma trigger. The problem is that asthma is not predictable, triggers are not always avoidable, and every time an episode occurs, the airways become more sensitive and reactive, more "twitchy." After a particularly severe episode it can take as long as a year for the lungs to return to normal. Having had this happen to me, I have reluctantly concluded that the best procedure is to use all available techniques—drugs, exercise, stress reduction, avoidance of triggers—to be as symptom-free as possible, in the hope that the twitchiness can be reduced to a minimum, and that it will eventually be practical to reduce dependence on medication. At present my attitude toward my inhaler is that I wouldn't leave home without it.

Self-care requires understanding the role of each medication you take and working with your doctor to ensure that the best possible results are being achieved. It also means being neither resistant to taking drugs nor totally dependent on them, but rather fitting them into an overall plan of maximum good health.

5

Adrenalin and Sympathomimetic (Adrenalin-like) Drugs

As we discussed in Chapter 4, "The Role of Asthma Medications," Adrenalin and sympathomimetic drugs stimulate the production of cAMP, a chemical in the lung's muscle cells that prevents bronchoconstriction. The sympathomimetic drugs function in the same way as Adrenalin but are more flexible because they can be taken orally or inhaled as well as given by injection. (The generic form of Adrenalin, epinephrine, is less familiar to most people than the trade name, so we will generally refer to Adrenalin from now on.) Because Adrenalin can be given only by injection, it is not likely to play a large part in self-management. The sympathomimetic drugs, however, will probably form the mainstay of your drug regimen.

Adrenalin and Adrenalin-like drugs that imitate the action of Adrenalin fall into the group known as beta-receptor-stimulating or beta-adrenergic drugs. They are bronchodilators, opening up the airways and restoring easy breathing; their special usefulness lies in their quick action. When you need relief fast, whether from mild discomfort or an acute attack, these sympathomimetic drugs are the drugs that you will probably reach for. They are all similar in action, side effects, speed of relief, and length of effectiveness; their differences are usually well known to the physician, who takes your entire health picture into account in choosing among them.

The sympathomimetic inhalers are the drugs of choice for pretreatment for exercise-induced asthma or bronchospasm. Since most of them are approved for use in sports competition worldwide, athletes with asthma tend to favor them. (Cromolyn sodium also is a good preventive asthma drug for pretreatment, but it has to build up in the system and, unlike the sympathomimetic drugs, cannot be taken on an as-needed or irregular basis; thus athletes who may not need a maintenance drug regimen are less likely to use it.)

Here are the some of the most commonly used drugs in this category.

Adrenalin

If you have gone to an emergency room with an asthmatic attack, you have probably been given an injection of Adrenalin as the initial treatment. If your attack is severe and does not respond sufficiently to the first injection within twenty minutes, you may be given a second Adrenalin injection. Chances are you will stop wheezing and begin to notice that you are feeling much better but shaky, with perhaps a tremor and a fast heartbeat. These side effects are normal reactions to Adrenalin and usually disappear fairly soon.

Although Adrenalin is not often self-administered, it is possible to give yourself an Adrenalin injection in an emergency. And it is especially useful for asthmatic travelers who may find themselves in a remote region far from conventional medical help. Your doctor can prescribe disposable Adrenalin kits to take with you, with instructions as to when and how to use them. Injecting yourself with these kits does not require any training or expertise, just an understanding of when to take this emergency measure.

A good way to keep Adrenalin on hand is the EpiPen, which is designed to deliver a single dose and is much easier to use than a standard hypodermic. A reduced-dose version, the EpiPen Jr., is available for children. EpiPen is only for emergency use and does not take the place of medical or hospital care, which should be sought as soon as possible after taking the medication.

If you have demonstrated a severe sensitivity to insect stings, food, or other allergens, with possible anaphylactic reactions, having an EpiPen handy may save your life. It can be stored at room temperature, so it is easy to take along when traveling.

EpiPen is available on prescription; ask your doctor about it and make careful notes of his or her instructions—when not to take it (it has some drug interactions), and especially how, where, and when to inject it.

Albuterol (Albutamol in Europe)

Available for inhaled, oral, and nebulizer use, albuterol (Proventil, Ventolin) is one of the most commonly prescribed inhaled asthma medications in this country. Its bronchodilating effect lasts from four to six hours, with little effect on the heart. In its oral forms, tablets and syrup, it sometimes causes a shaky feeling.

Bitolterol

Bitolterol (Tornalate) is a new inhaled bronchodilator. Whereas the albuterol inhalers contain two hundred "puffs," Tornalate contains three hundred. It is longer-lasting than isoproterenol (see below) and may be effective for five to eight hours.

Ephedrine

Fifteen years ago this was often the drug of choice for patient use, and it is still the only oral sympathomimetic drug cleared by the FDA for use during pregnancy. It was often taken (and is still available) as a combination drug in oral form, such as Marax and Tedral tablets, which also contain theophylline and phenobarbital.

Ephedrine acts quickly and works well for some people but not for others. It tends to make you feel very shaky and tremulous (in spite of the sedative, which is meant to alleviate that feeling but is not desirable for asthmatics) and may increase blood pressure and cause insomnia.

Some physicians do not recommend it for a number of reasons and feel there are better, more sophisticated drugs available. The theophylline component of the tablets is fixed and does not allow for the variation in dosage that current medical practice prefers. And phenobarbital is not generally recommended for asthmatics. Also, some brands (such as Tedral) are sold as over-the-counter (OTC) drugs in many states, and many physicians feel that increases the possibility of its being used inappropriately or even too casually for such a powerful medication.

Older asthmatics who used Tedral and similar combinations before some of the other drugs were available still sometimes keep them on hand and swear nothing else is as effective when the symptoms are very uncomfortable. This kind of combination drug is available in tablets, sustained-action (SA) tablets, and a syrup.

Isoetharine

Isoetharine (Bronkometer, Bronkosol) is similar to isoproterenol but a weaker bronchodilator, with less untoward effect on the heart. Bronkosol contains acetone sodium bisulfite, which can cause serious side effects in someone sensitive to sulfites.

Isoproterenol (Isoprenalin in Europe)

Isoproterenol is an inhaled bronchodilator found in both prescription (Medihaler-Iso, Duo-Medihaler, Isuprel Mistometer) and over-the-counter forms. Isuprel also comes in tablet form and for nebulizers. It acts quickly but is of comparatively short duration (about two hours inhaled), which has led to decreased use, although it is still sometimes used in the emergency room instead of Adrenalin.

Metaproterenol

Metaproterenol (Alupent, Metaprel) is available as an inhaler and as tablets or syrup. Alupent also comes as a liquid for the nebulizer. Metaproterenol is popular with some physicians because of a tendency to less stimulation of the heart; others prefer albuterol or terbutaline because they act more directly on the lungs.

Don't Take Asthma for Granted

A visit to the emergency room may be a sign that something has gone wrong with your control, and events leading up to the attack should be reviewed to see whether you can prevent it from happening again. Whenever your symptoms start to get worse, and the medication and techniques you are supposed to use are not helping, it is important not to delay seeking medical help, either from your physician or in the emergency room (which may be quicker).

Once the emergency has been dealt with, try to figure out what happened to cause the asthma to get out of your control. If the attack was due to a reaction to a bee sting, ingestion of a sulfite, or some other particularly strong-reacting trigger, you can only try to avoid the trigger in the future and possibly keep an EpiPen or similar injectible, quick-response medication on hand for unavoidable encounters. Most of the time, however, worsening asthma probably crept up on you without your realizing it, or you overestimated your ability to deal with it.

The better the job you have been doing, or the longer you have had asthma, the more likely you are to become overconfident, complacent, or simply accepting of a certain amount of discomfort. Using a peak-flow meter regularly will give you an unbiased reading of your condition and help you to spot a downward trend that you might not otherwise be aware of. The few minutes a day it takes can prevent you from losing days or weeks in a hospital.

Terbutaline

Terbutaline (Brethaire, Brethine, Bricanyl) varies in form according to brand. Brethaire comes only in an MDI (metered-dose inhaler—see pages 76–77); Brethine and Bricanyl come in oral and injectable form. It is quick-acting, and the effect may last for four to eight hours.

Why Do Drugs Come in So Many Different Forms?

The variations of form offer the physician great flexibility in setting up a course of treatment. For instance, they make it possible, where the drugs are compatible, to prescribe two different drugs, one as an inhalant, the other as a tablet; a Ventolin inhaler, for example, may be backed up by a maintenance schedule of Brethine. Many asthmatics have both an inhaler and an oral medication as their maintenance regime. Often the relationship is synergistic, with the combination working better than each drug taken alone. (This is not why inhaled steroids are also added to the treatment; their function is preventive and does not relate to these other drugs except insofar as all try, by various methods, to control asthma symptoms.)

6

Theophylline

In the United States, for the past thirty years, theophylline has been the single most widely prescribed oral asthma medication. Because of this, it has paid the pharmaceutical manufacturers to provide it in many forms, and so it is exceptionally "user-friendly," not only in the form of tablets, including chewable tablets, but also as capsules, liquids, and syrups. In addition to regular capsules, theophylline comes in capsules such as Slo-Bid and Theo-Dur Sprinkle. In this form the capsule contains "beads" designed to be sprinkled on a spoonful of some soft food, such as applesauce or pudding, which should then be swallowed immediately, followed by water or juice to make sure the entire dose has gone down. (It is important that the food be soft because the beads should not be chewed, and care should be taken that neither the food nor the liquid is hot.) Sprinkles, like syrups, are designed for children and adults who have trouble swallowing medication.

Theophylline is not available as an inhalant, but in a different form, such as aminophylline, it is sometimes given intravenously, either by syringe or infusion, when immediate relief is required. Infusion is usually the method of choice, since theophylline must be introduced slowly (instructions for syringe injection always emphasize that it must be given very, very slowly).

Theophylline comes in different strengths, from 50 mg. to 500 mg. Sometimes you have occasion to take half a dose, but unless the tablet you have is scored to be broken in half, do not break it or powder it. (Half of a nonscored tablet may not contain half a dose.) It also comes four ways: short-acting, intermediate-acting, long-acting, and twenty-four-hour-acting. If your asthma is mild and you need medication only occasionally, the short-acting, which peaks in two hours and can be taken every four hours, will probably be sufficient. Long-acting, on the other hand, is usually prescribed for chronic or severe asthma, and its effectiveness depends on cumulatively reaching an ideal serum level. Once that level has been established, the drug should be taken regularly, usually every twelve hours, so as to maintain it.

The ability to prescribe theophylline in so many different ways is especially helpful to the physician because there is a comparatively small margin between an effective dose and one that is toxic. Too little will be ineffectual; too much can be fatal. Establishing the right dosage for a patient is complicated by the fact that different individuals metabolize theophylline at different rates. One person may reach a therapeutically effective level on a dose that is totally ineffective for another.

Not only do absorption and metabolism rates vary from person to person but also certain personal habits—such as whether an asthmatic smokes (tobacco or marijuana)—and diet preferences affect theophylline blood serum levels.

There is now a simple blood test, which can be done in the doctor's office less expensively than having it done by a lab, that indicates whether you are getting the correct dosage. If at any time you feel you are not getting sufficient relief, let your doctor know. He or she will probably do this test before increasing the dose appreciably.

The Caffeine Connection

Theophylline is related to caffeine, found in colas, cocoa, coffee, and tea (tea contains actual theophylline as well). If you are a coffee or tea drinker, you may be pleased to know that a hot cup of your favorite beverage can be medically therapeutic as well as pleasurable, and an ice-cold cola drink on a hot day may do more than refresh. None of these can be counted on for anything like the degree of relief of your theophylline prescription, but if you don't have medication handy, a cup or two of strong, hot tea or coffee might contribute, however slightly, to making you more comfortable.

On the other hand, since these beverages increase the theophyllinelike substances in your system, drinking quantities of them may create side effects. It is not advisable to use them to help swallow theophylline tablets. And if you tend to consume any of them in large quantities—such as several cups of coffee a day—check with your doctor as to whether this is safe.

If you are on theophylline and experience unusual shakiness or jitteriness after drinking or eating, make a note of what you have ingested, and if it happens again, tell your doctor.

Furthermore, when going for a serum theophylline test, be sure to tell the doctor if you have had coffee, cocoa, tea, a cola drink, chocolate, or acetaminophen (such as Tylenol) less than an hour before; any of these might invalidate the test results.

How Theophylline Works

Theophylline is thought to act directly on the smooth muscles of the bronchial tubes as a bronchodilator. When these muscles contract, they narrow the airways and cause bronchospasm; theophylline, by relaxing these muscles, opens the airways and relieves the asthma. In addition, it prevents the release of bronchoconstricting chemicals, such as histamine.

Theophylline differs from other bronchodilators, such as albuterol, in that it is not indicated when you are actually having an attack. If you are experiencing uncomfortable shortness of breath, what you need is a drug that will work right away; even short-acting theophylline takes effect too slowly to be helpful then.

Side Effects

If the dose is right, any side effects felt initially will tend to disappear as the body adjusts to the theophylline. The most common side effects are mild nausea, rapid heartbeat, slight shakiness, and irritability, but these are not invariably experienced. Another possible side effect may be more frequent urination, since theophylline can act as a mild diuretic. You should be aware, however, that it is possible for more serious side effects to occur without warning and in the absence of milder side effects. Vomiting, a bad headache, unusual shakiness, or palpitations and fast heartbeat may signal an overdose. Since this can happen inadvertently (for example, if you develop a heart or liver problem, make an extreme change in your diet, or get a viral infection), it is important to report any reactions to your doctor and let him or her evaluate them. So many things—even an influenza immunization injection—can cause a change in serum theophylline clearance that it is not practical for you to try to deal with side effects. Only a serum theophylline test can determine what is really occurring in your system, and only a doctor can deal with it.

Because of the potential seriousness of a theophylline overdose, no side effects, whatever the cause, should be ignored, and extremely unpleasant ones should receive immediate, emergency room–type attention. Observation, not apprehension, is the key: do not anticipate that you will be troubled by side effects, simply be aware of the possibility. Given the wide use and effectiveness of theophylline, it is obvious that it is generally prescribed successfully and is a safe and useful medication. Your job as the manager of your asthma is to recognize any unusual reactions and seek appropriate help.

Occasionally a person may simply not be able to tolerate the effective dose of theophylline (just as some asthmatics cannot tolerate aspirin) and will need to discontinue it completely. This does not happen very often, and when it does, other medications are available to replace the theophylline.

It is possible to have an adverse reaction to almost any new drug or treatment, but simple observation of yourself should alert you to the need for professional advice. In every instance, remember, it is always better to seek help and find you did not really need it than to wait too long to take remedial action.

Diet and Other Factors That Affect Theophylline Absorption

Since the rate at which theophylline is metabolized is so critical, given the somewhat narrow margin between an effective dose and an overdose, it is no surprise that what enters your body as food, drink, or other ingested or inhaled substances can affect the dosage of the medication. Depending on the substance that is introduced into the system, the elimination of theophylline can be either speeded up or slowed; both are undesirable. The first means that serum theophylline is not maintained at an effective level and fails to provide the needed relief. The second results in a cumulative buildup of serum theophylline as the previous dose, not properly eliminated, combines with the next dose; the result, given the narrow margin of safety, can be an overdose.

Among the foods that affect serum theophylline metabolism, some studies have indicated, is the traditional American steak-and-potatoes diet, which is high in protein and fat and low in carbohydrates and may possibly speed the elimination of theophylline by as much as 25 percent. If, on the other hand, you are a vegetarian or, in keeping with modern dietary guidelines, have adopted a a low-protein, low-fat, high-carbohydrate diet, the dosage adjustment will be somewhat different, since absorption may be slowed by a like percentage. Much more research is needed to confirm this possibility, but if this is your usual diet and your theophylline doesn't seem to be working as well as expected, your dosage may have to be adjusted.

It is probably a good idea to try to maintain your normal diet pattern, whatever it is, once your effective theophylline level has been established. Then, if no other unusual lifestyle changes occur, that level should tend to stay within the same range. Of course, if you suddenly increase your daily intake of coffee or colas, or go on a new medication that reacts with theophylline, your doctor should be notified.

Generally speaking, the most asked question, "Should theophylline be taken with food?" cannot be answered definitively at this time. The effect of food intake on the drug is still being studied and has not been determined. To date, according to the manufacturer, it does not seem to matter whether you take Theo-Dur before, after, or between meals. Some doctors think, however, that while it may be more effective when taken on an empty stomach, it is more liable to cause digestive problems; they tend to recommend that you take it after a meal. The important thing is consistency; whenever you take it, try to do so under the same conditions (before a meal, after a meal) each time.

As we have already noted, smoking affects theophylline metabolism; just one pack a day sharply speeds the rate at which it is eliminated. A further problem for smokers is that it may take as long as two years after cessation of smoking for the body's metabolism of theophylline to return to normal. Alcoholism has the opposite effect and can be doubly serious in the presence of already impaired kidney function, which in itself slows the elimination of theophylline. Certain other illnesses, such as congestive heart failure and COPD (chronic obstructive pulmonary disease), may increase the usual half-life, and elderly patients often metabolize theophylline more slowly than those under age fifty-five.

As long as you are consistent in your habits, whether dietary

---

Generic Theophylline

Although the generic equivalents of most prescription drugs, when available, are less expensive and therefore desirable if the doctor has no objection to them, theophylline is an exception; it is generally thought that taking the generic form of theophylline is not a good idea. If your doctor agrees, his prescriptions for specific theophylline drugs should carry a note for the pharmacist: "Do not substitute."

or smoking, your doctor will automatically adjust the dosage to what you as an individual seem to require as indicated by the serum level tests. It would be better if he or she knew what was causing you to vary from the norm, but it is not absolutely essential in these instances. It doesn't hurt, however, for you to be aware of the influence these factors have, so that if you change your habits, you have a clue when your theophylline dosage seems to suddenly become less—or more—effective. If that should occur and you suspect you know the reason, share it with your doctor; the more information he has, the better he can do his job.

There are, however, factors beyond your control, which may change your metabolism of theophylline. Illness, especially a viral illness with accompanying fever, may slow elimination, leading to a possible overdose. Be sure to tell your doctor if you think you have a viral illness—certainly, if you have any significant fever.

Theophylline and Drug Interactions

As with any new regimen, be sure your doctor is aware of any other drugs you may be taking or ones you add on subsequently. If you are being treated by an allergist or pulmonary specialist, you may not think to mention drugs already prescribed by your internist, cardiologist, dentist, or other doctors. Over-the-counter drugs are often overlooked, but all of them should also be mentioned to your doctor. All drugs have their own peculiar effects on the system and may interact with any new ones that are suddenly introduced. Even if all you are taking is something you routinely use, like a sedative, bring in a complete list, with the size and frequency of the dose you are taking.

Among the drugs with which theophylline interacts are cimetidine (Tagamet) and the antibiotics erythromycin and troleandomycin, which increase the absorption of theophylline and therefore may require a decrease in your usual theophylline dose during the time you are on them. It also interacts with propranolol (Inderal) by antagonizing or inhibiting its effects. Lithium, on the other hand, is enhanced by theophylline, and therefore the size of the lithium dose needs to be considered.

Beta-Stimulating Drugs (Beta-Agonists)

Another group of medications that may increase theophylline absorption are known as beta-stimulating drugs. These drugs include such inhalants as albuterol, bitolterol, isoetharine, and terbutaline (some are also available in tablet form). There are indications that a synergistic relationship exists with this group. Since they are drugs often included, along with theophylline, in asthma management programs, such a relationship would be important and helpful if established.

It would then require a lower dose of theophylline and a beta-agonist in combination to achieve the same effect as a higher dose of either one taken alone. And since they are so often used together for long-term, ongoing asthma management, it is especially desirable to be able to take the smallest possible dose. In any event, if your asthma seems to be more and more under control, your doctor will probably lower the doses even if he or she does not know why improvement is occurring—so you may benefit from the combination working this way in your case.

Aminophylline

If you have an episode that requires a visit to an emergency room, you will probably be given oxygen and an injection of Adrenalin. If this is not sufficient to reverse the bronchospasm, you may subsequently be given aminophylline, which is 85 percent anhydrous theophylline (the kind of theophylline in Theo-Dur), intravenously. If you ask what you have been given, you may be told simply "theophylline," which is basically accurate.

Since, as noted earlier in this chapter, intravenous aminophylline must be given very slowly (too rapid a delivery is liable to cause dangerously unpleasant reactions), it is now more commonly delivered with an IV drip. If, however, you should have an injection, do not be impatient if the procedure seems to be taking an inordinately long time.

Other forms in which aminophylline is available are rectal suppositories, rectal enemas, tablets, and liquid.

Theophylline in Combination with Other Drugs

Originally theophylline was made in the form of tablets that contained various other drugs; as mentioned, a popular brand, Tedral, contains ephedrine and phenobarbital as well as theophylline. While still available, combination drugs are no longer widely prescribed because physicians prefer the flexibility of theophylline-only preparations. Given the wide range of individual metabolism rates of theophylline, the physician prefers the option of adjusting the dose to each patient's needs. A patient who requires more theophylline, for instance, would have to take more tablets, thus also getting more phenobarbital and ephedrine, which would not necessarily be needed.

There is no doubt, however, that Tedral can sometimes give quick relief when the inhaler does not, and patients who have had Tedral prescribed in the past sometimes continue to use an occasional tablet as a backup. Your doctor may prefer, however, that you use a noncombination short-acting theophylline tablet or some other medication as a backup.

Again, it is not wise to ever prescribe for yourself or to change your doctor's instructions. If you find yourself reaching for medications outside your established regimen, check with your doctor as to whether that is advisable or whether he or she would prefer some other drug instead. This applies especially to over-the-counter (OTC) preparations, which are difficult for the layman to evaluate and may be inappropriate for your situation.

How to Take Theophylline

Your doctor will probably suggest which form (tablets, capsules, sprinkles, or other) is most suitable. If you have trouble swallowing capsules or even tablets, let him or her know. Do not powder the tablets or open the capsules without asking whether this is all right with the type of theophylline prescribed.

Long-acting and Short-acting Theophylline

From the patient's point of view, the difference between the short- and long-acting theophylline is threefold; relief, convenience, and consistency. The short-acting form will bring immediate relief while the long-acting takes longer to work. On the other hand, the short-acting has to be taken twice as often and may have more ups and downs of the serum theophylline level with a shorter relief span. For example, short-acting theophylline, which is taken every six hours, is primarily useful for asthmatics who are free of symptoms most of the time, with only occasional asthma. This type usually comes in capsule form, although at least one brand makes chewable tablets, and short-acting theophylline liquid is also available.

Long-acting theophylline is taken every twelve hours and tends to maintain a more even serum theophylline level. In addition, the morning dose means minimum interference with the day's activities, while the evening dose increases the likelihood of a good night's sleep. The long-acting type is also handy for children, since it reduces the necessity of more frequent monitoring.

The chief disadvantage of the long-acting type is that those who metabolize theophylline quickly may find that their serum theophylline level drops too far before the next dose is indicated, with the result that their asthma is imperfectly controlled.

In practice, inhaled bronchodilators such as albuterol are used more frequently than theophylline to provide quick relief because of their shorter reaction time, while theophylline is usually taken, as additional medication, as part of a stabilizing maintenance program. An example of this would be a Ventolin inhaler, with one or two puffs every four hours or as needed, combined with a Theo-Dur tablet twice a day.

The Changing Use of Theophylline

Although statistically theophylline is still the leader in asthma medications, there seems to be a growing trend toward phasing it out in favor of some of the newer drugs. Europe has long since discarded it as a primary drug and relies much more heavily, for instance, on Intal. In addition, as you will see in the final chapter, prevention, rather than control, of symptoms seems to be the new approach.

7

The Pros and Cons of Corticosteroids

There are several types of steroids, but the ones used in the treatment of asthma are corticosteroids, synthetic adrenocortical steroids derived from cortisol, a natural hormone produced by the adrenal gland. Corticosteroids are available in various forms: as inhalants, tablets, suppositories, and liquid for injection. You will most often encounter them as inhalants or tablets. They are commonly referred to simply as steroids.

Corticosteroids are powerful anti-inflammatory drugs that reduce allergic reactions by inhibiting the formation and release of eosinophils (white blood cells that cause inflammation) and by relaxing airway constriction and in general alleviating asthma symptoms. As noted above, the steroids prescribed for asthma are usually given in one of two forms, oral and inhaled. As we will see, there is some difference in their action, particularly in the side effects.

Steroids as Muscle Builders ───

People are sometimes concerned, when their doctor prescribes steroids, that taking the drug will give them bulging, oversized muscles. There is no need to worry; there are many different steroids, and the kind prescribed for asthma is entirely different from the kind sometimes used by athletes.

Technically, the steroids used to treat asthma are adrenocorticoids, a synthetic version of a type of steroid produced by the adrenal glands. The particular corticosteroids, as they are sometimes referred to, used for asthma are glucocorticoids, but all you need to know is the term "steroids."

What athletes and bodybuilders sometimes use to try to build muscle are anabolic steroids. These steroids are usually banned in athletics, and although they, too, are referred to simply as steroids in the sports pages, they are entirely different from the steroids prescribed for asthma. When the subject is asthma medication, the term "steroids" always refers to a potent anti-inflammatory drug legally prescribed for the treatment of respiratory diseases.

Oral Steroids

In tablet (oral) form (for example, Prednisone, Prednisolone, Medrol) steroids are used primarily when other medications are failing to control the asthma. A short course of steroids is often sufficient to halt the acute phase of an attack and to make it possible for other medications to take over again. Long-term use of steroids is avoided as much as possible because of their undesirable side effects.

How They Work

The first effect of oral steroids on acute asthma is dramatic. You will feel more comfortable very quickly; airway constriction will lessen as muscles relax, much less mucus will be produced, and you will breathe easier in a very short time. The first time you experience the effect of an oral steroid on your asthma, your reaction is likely to be: "Why can't I use this all the time?" Unfortunately, the trade-off is that the possible side effects from any long-term use are numerous and possibly serious. For short-term use, though, there is nothing like it.

The second, longer-lasting effect occurs more slowly. Control of the asthma symptoms is maintained, usually preventing further attacks. Ideally, this maintenance function gives the body time to calm down so that other medications once again become effective. This, however, is achieved at a price.

Oral steroids work the same way the natural steroids produced by your body do, but there is one important difference: they can be given in amounts greater than that which your body normally produces. The amount prescribed and the length of time over which they are taken vary, depending on the severity of the asthma. Do not attempt to medicate yourself with steroids, even if you have some left over from an earlier prescription. Steroids should be taken only with a doctor's direction and supervision.

Unfortunately, the body can't tell the difference between its own product and the synthetic steroid drug you are taking. As a result, it is liable to note that the amount of steroid in your system is now sufficient—probably more than it is programmed to produce—and therefore it reduces or even shuts down its own production. Since naturally produced steroids are extremely important to the functioning of your body, the physician always takes care to try not to decrease your normal production any more, or for any longer, than is strictly necessary to control asthma symptoms. Restoring the body's own production to normal levels is tricky and, again, must always be managed by a doctor. Never decide you know how to do it on your own.

There are a number of ways the doctor can minimize inhibiting your body's own production of steroids. The first is to prescribe as low a dose for as short a time as is needed to be effective. This will vary with your rate of metabolism, the severity of your asthma, and other individual factors.

Many physicians favor an every-other-day program that, when it is appropriate, allows your body a recovery period in between. The theory is that on the days you are not taking your tablets your body will produce its own steroids and normal production will continue without interruption.

Another variable is the time of day when the steroids are taken. There are two schools of thought. Since the body's own steroid production tends to peak in early morning, you may be told to take your entire day's dose at breakfast, which is closest to the body's natural timing and presumably least inhibits natural production. Some doctors, on the other hand, prefer to stagger the dosage so that you take it three or four times during the day. Whatever schedule you are on, follow it faithfully, taking the tablets at the same time every day.

The size of the dosage will vary according to the severity of your asthma and how effective steroids are in controlling your symptoms. There is considerable variation among patients and also from incident to incident, but the effort is always to achieve the lowest possible effective dose over the shortest possible time. The ability to prescribe different strengths and frequency of dosages gives the doctor a great deal of leeway, and the more familiar he or she becomes with you and your reactions to various drugs, the easier it will be to prescribe for your individual needs.

If you are given a schedule for a week or ten days and then, after checking with the doctor, are told to repeat the program, do not assume that it is not working, or that the doctor should have given you a stronger dose the first time. Most doctors will try to prescribe steroids conservatively. They would rather repeat the prescription a second time, or even increase the dose for the second schedule, than initially give you more than you need.

Your observations and report on how you are progressing is critical. Always check with the doctor promptly upon completion of a course of steroids and be prepared to report either improvement or the lack of it.

Winding Down a Steroid Prescription

An important part of a steroid prescription is the winding-down period, when you start decreasing the dosage. This has to be done fairly slowly so that the body has time to note and send signals to your adrenal gland that there is now a deficiency to be made up and body production needs to be reactivated or increased. Since it takes at least three days for the adrenal gland to respond and gear up production after even a comparatively short course of steroids, and since you would not want to find yourself without an adequate supply in your system, the winding-down period is as important as the rest of the schedule. When you are down to one tablet a day, it is just as important to take it on schedule as when you were taking several.

The longer you have been on steroids, the longer it will take for your own production to resume; it can be as long as six months if you have been on steroids for an extended treatment.

Fortunately, there are more and more ways to decrease the need for oral steroids. Inhaled steroids can often replace or reduce the need for oral, once the asthma is somewhat under control, and medications are currently being developed that may replace them or at least reduce the occasions when they are needed. Even status asthmaticus, where steroids are part of the treatment, calls for theophylline and other maintenance medications (though in increased dosages) in the regime. Like fire, steroids are a good servant but a bad master and require close medical supervision to enhance the good and minimize the bad.

When Oral Steroids Are Used

Because of possibly serious side effects, oral steroids are primarily used as a last resort when other medications fail to control the asthma. At present there is almost nothing to take their place, and when they are used properly, side effects can often be minimized. Unfortunately, less experienced physicians may sometimes use them longer and stronger than is desirable, in a desperate last-ditch effort to help the patient.

In discussions with physicians at the National Jewish Center for Immunology and Respiratory Medicine, I asked a number of them, "What is the first problem you encounter with patients coming to the Center from other physicians?" The answer almost invariably was "Weaning them off oral steroids." Since most patients end up at National Jewish because their asthma has become chronically severe and unmanageable and can no longer be controlled by their own physicians, this situation is not surprising. What is surprising, and encouraging, is that the Center's doctors are frequently able to either reduce the dose or even discontinue it entirely through their treatments and regime.

This is not to say that you should automatically resist taking oral steroids when your doctor prescribes them. They can be literally lifesaving and are appropriate treatment when nothing else is working. Almost all asthmatics will be grateful for their help at certain times.

Incidentally, the body's reaction to inhaled steroids is thought to be quite different, as we will see later on in this chapter.

Advantages of Oral Steroids

Oral steroids work when other medication does not. They can not only prevent attacks, they can also reverse them and allow time for twitchy airways to calm down and respond to other medications. In an emergency room situation an epinephrine injection is usually the first medication given, but under home conditions, for troublesome but less severe episodes, a course of oral steroids will often do the trick. Regular use of a peak-flow meter should alert you to increased asthma and give you ample time to call your doctor so he or she can temporarily increase your maintenance medication or possibly add the oral steroids, thus avoiding a visit to the emergency room.

(Sometimes, however, the latter is the best choice. While no one wants to go to an emergency room, there are times when it is the only sensible thing to do and the best way to avoid getting so out of control as to require hospitalization. You should talk to your doctor about this when setting up your maintenance schedule so you know the most appropriate action to take when your regular asthma worsens.)

Side Effects of Oral Steroids

Side effects are not inevitable, nor does everyone experience them, and those from short-term use often clear up as soon as medication is discontinued. The most serious side effects occur only after years of use. But since you are in control of your own asthma, you will want to know what they are.

Weight Gain   The side effects that are most quickly noticed are increased appetite and weight gain. Your face may become puffy, and if you retain water, your ankles and feet may swell.

The best way to deal with weight gain is to go on a diet, following the usual rules for losing weight. High-fiber, low-fat foods, more carbohydrates than protein, low-calorie snacks (carrots instead of candy), and low sodium intake will all help. You may still find it difficult to control some weight gain, but at least you can be sure that once you discontinue the steroids, you will be able to get back to your normal weight fairly easily. If steroid use lasts only a week or two, you probably won't have this problem. (Just don't keep on eating after your appetite has returned to normal.)

If the weight gain is due to water retention, a prescription diuretic will help.

If it is a long-term course of steroids and weight gain is a problem, discuss it with your physician.

Indigestion   Steroid tablets may upset your stomach, sometimes to the point of causing stomach ulcers. To minimize this, always take them with food. A glass of milk is sufficient, but you can generally coordinate your schedule so that you take the tablets at a regular mealtime.

If you get indigestion, an antacid may help. Any extreme discomfort should be reported.

Nutritional Deficiencies   Sometimes long-term or frequent use of oral steroids will cause a potassium or calcium deficiency. Diuretics may also cause a potassium deficiency. Bananas and citrus fruits are good sources of potassium, and most of us already know about calcium sources. If in doubt, pick up one of the many inexpensive paperbacks dealing with vitamins and minerals.

Cataracts and Glaucoma   Steroids seem to increase the incidence of cataracts and may also cause glaucoma. Tell your ophthalmologist if you are on long-term oral steroids, and ask how often he thinks you should have a checkup. Cataracts start small and usually develop slowly, finally making themselves felt in vision changes, but glaucoma can sneak up on you and do irreversible damage if not treated.

Skin Problems   Ironically, although steroids in the form of over-the-counter hydrocortisone creams and ointments are used in the treatment of many skin conditions, oral steroids can occasionally cause acne.

You may also notice that, due to thinning of the skin, you bruise more easily and even minor scratches and bruises seem to heal more slowly.

There may be a slight increase in facial hair, but it will be very fine and is not usually a problem.

Fortunately, all these side effects tend to be reversible.

Infections   Oral steroids depress the immune system, which makes you more vulnerable to infections and less able to fight them. When you are actively taking steroids, and for a week or two after, try to avoid crowds. Dinner parties, going to the movies, even visiting a nursing home or attending a lecture, are all events that may expose you to colds, the flu, and similar infections. If in spite of precautions you do get an infection of any sort, mention it to your doctor.

Osteoporosis   Although osteoporosis is primarily a disease that afflicts the elderly, it is also, unfortunately, liable to be caused at any age by long-term use of oral steroids. The thinning and demineralization of the bone that characterizes osteoporosis increases the possibility of fractures, even under only moderately stressful conditions. For example, the frequent occurrence of broken hips in older people is due to osteoporosis. Although generally considered irreversible in the elderly, drug-induced osteoporosis appears to be reversible in children and even in young adults.

At present there is no cure, but there is some evidence that vitamin and mineral supplements may help. Since this is a comparatively new area, ask your doctor or respiratory therapist, or if they do not seem to be knowledgeable about it, talk to a nutritionist. Do not attempt to prescribe for yourself by reading about vitamins and nutritional supplements, because here you are dealing with a medical problem, not a dietary deficiency, and may end up with severe side effects from overdoing the supplement doses. Asthmatics with osteoporosis due to long-term steroid use are under sufficient stress without subjecting themselves to the possible dangers of this type of self-medication.

Retarded Growth   When steroids are needed to control childhood asthma, it is especially important to use them judiciously and for as short a time as possible. Long-term oral steroid use in children can cause irreversible growth retardation. The effectiveness of steroids, however, means that sometimes they are the drug of choice in spite of their side effects. Severe asthma needs to be gotten under control as soon as possible, whether in child or adult, and in such a situation the benefits of steroids far outweigh the disadvantages.

Mood Changes   Long-term use, over a period of years for example, can cause noticeable mood changes. Almost everyone experiences a feeling of euphoria when first taking steroids; aside from anything else, the relief from asthma is enough to make one feel good. But the mood change in long-term use is just the opposite; the patient may become very depressed or irritable, and sometimes the personality change is serious enough to suggest the need for therapy. Since the patient may not be aware of this kind of symptom, it is important for family and close friends to be alert to the possibility, and the doctor should be notified if such a side effect is suspected.

Thrush   Oral steroids, as well as inhaled steroids, may cause thrush infections (see page 59). This is more likely to happen with large doses or long courses, and to diabetics.

Headaches   Since so many things can cause headaches, it may be difficult to connect a headache with the taking of oral steroids. If, however, you have headaches infrequently and notice that you have them more often when on oral steroids, there may be a connection. This is not likely to be a severe problem but should be mentioned to your doctor if you think the drug is the cause.

Leg Cramps   Usually leg cramps due to steroids will not be severe. If you are bothered by them upon awakening in the morning, take an extra moment in bed to stretch your legs. Lie flat on your back and flex your feet at right angles to your legs. Then push your legs forward and back alternately a few times, bending your knees slightly. This will often loosen your calf muscles and relieve the cramps. If it is going to work, it will do so immediately and can stop even a fairly severe cramp.

Leg cramps are often caused by having the bedclothes tucked in too tightly. Be sure they are loosened over your feet, and do not press your toes down toward the bottom sheet; anything that forces your feet into this position may cause leg cramps. Lying on your side will also reduce pressure on your toes.

A potassium deficiency can cause leg cramps that will disappear when the diet is adjusted. Orange juice and bananas, among many other foods, are fairly high in potassium. If the problem persists, see your doctor.

Increased Blood Sugar   Unless you are a diabetic, an increase in blood sugar due to oral steroids generally is not a cause for concern, but it is well to be aware of this possible side effect.

Increased Blood Pressure   Because steroids have a tendency to increase salt and therefore water retention, they may cause an increase in your blood pressure, but that is easy to monitor, and your doctor undoubtedly checks each time he sees you. Since high blood pressure is symptomless and you have no way of telling if you have it, you should keep this side effect in mind. If you have been taking oral steroids for some months without needing an office visit, you can still arrange to drop in just for a blood pressure check or, if handier, probably get your blood pressure checked at the district nurse's office or local community health center (they usually have regular times for doing this). Ask your doctor how often he or she advises a blood pressure check in your case.

Inhaled Steroids

Use of inhaled steroids (for example, Vanceril, Azmacort, Aero-Bid) has increased considerably in recent years, because of a greater understanding of the role inflammation plays in triggering asthma attacks. Unlike the tablets, inhaled steroids are usually incorporated into routine maintenance regimes to prevent inflammation. As far as is known at this time, they do not have the undesirable side effects of other forms of steroids; one of the very few they may have is thrush (see below), which is generally easily prevented by carefully rinsing the mouth and gargling with plain warm water immediately after use.

How to Take Inhaled Steroids

Since inhaled steroids are not bronchodilators, they should always be preceded by two puffs (at least five minutes apart) from an inhaled bronchodilator. This serves to open the airways so that as much of the steroid as possible gets as deeply as possible into the lungs. Obviously, inhaled steroids are useless during an acute asthma attack, since the constricted airways prevent the medication from getting deeply enough into the problem area. What is needed at that juncture is a bronchodilator.

To minimize the frequency with which you have to think about medication and to make it easier to remember to take them, coordinate inhaled steroids with your regular inhaled broncho-

dilator schedule. For instance, if you use the inhaled bronchodilator regularly morning and evening (in addition to any other
times), use the inhaled steroid at the same time (if it is prescribed
for twice a day). Generally, you will use inhaled steroids twice a
day.

Inhaled steroids come two ways: for puffing into the mouth
and for spraying into the nose. Often both are prescribed. If you
use an inhaled nasal steroid (Vancenase, Beconase, Nasalide,
Decadron, beclomethasone, flunisolide) in addition to a steroid
inhaler, use the nasal right after the inhaled mouth steroid; a
waiting period between mouth steroid puffs is not necessary.
Then rinse and gargle only one time for both steroids.

Incidentally, if you have allergies and have had to suffer with
stuffy nose and congested sinuses, you will find the nasal steroids
very helpful in keeping your head clear.

Inhaled nasal steroids are not used to mitigate an asthma
attack; their function is preventive.

Advantages of Inhaled Steroids

Far fewer side effects occur with inhaled (as compared to
oral) steroids. As we have seen, aside from thrush, none of the
side effects usually associated with steroid use have been noted.
This means that inhaled steroids can be used as long as necessary
and can be incorporated with bronchodilators in a regular, ongoing maintenance program. Increased control of asthma symptoms results, as well as a reduction in asthma flares.

It is thought that there are fewer side effects because the
inhaled steroid does not go through the body and into the bloodstream but is instead delivered directly to the site (the airways
and the lungs). You will not, for instance, get a puffy face or
increased appetite from nasal steroids.

Regular use of inhaled steroids may reduce the need for oral
steroids, making it possible to decrease the size of the oral dose.

Side Effects of Inhaled Steroids

Thrush   As noted above, inhaled steroids can cause the formation of thrush. This is a fungus infection that shows up as white patches on mucous membranes; it is easy to spot with even a cursory examination of the mouth and back of the throat. Since it often doesn't cause any discomfort, regularly examine your mouth: lift up your tongue and look at the back of your throat, using a flashlight if necessary. If you haven't been in the habit of doing this, you may mistake a coated tongue for thrush. Check with your doctor if you are not sure, and let him or her decide what it is. If it is thrush, the doctor may temporarily reduce your steroid dose or prescribe a special medicated gargle to clear up the fungus.

Light Local Nose Bleeding   Occasionally nasal inhaled steroids may cause bleeding (noticeable when you blow your nose) or tenderness in the nose. If that should happen, tell your doctor. He or she may advise decreasing the frequency of the nasal spray for a while or using nasal lavage to soothe the lining. This is not a symptom to ignore, but it is not serious.

Hoarseness   You may not immediately associate this symptom with inhaled steroids, but it is a fairly common reaction. Tell your doctor as soon as you notice it. A short rest from steroid medication will usually cause the condition to disappear, but do not discontinue your regimen on your own; let your doctor manage this end of it.

Steroids and Drug Interactions

With a chronic disease sooner or later a problem arises about possible interactions between the drugs prescribed for that disease and drugs taken for other health conditions. This is true of steroids as well as other asthma medications. Although you cannot possibly know the specifics firsthand, you can be aware that there may be a problem and check it out whenever you start to take a new drug; this is important with over-the-counter drugs— which you may take on your own—as well as prescription drugs.

Barbiturates, ephedrine, and some antibiotics (such as rifampin) speed up the metabolism of steroids. This means that if you are taking a steroid at the same time as any of these drugs, the steroid dose will have a greater effect (since the body is absorbing it more quickly), and the effect will not last as long (because it is used up faster). The opposite—a slowing down of steroid metabolism—occurs with a number of other antibiotics, with estrogen, and with cromolyn sodium.

Either reaction requires an adjustment in the steroid dose from what you would normally need. Thus doctors must know what other drugs you are taking. And it is up to you to provide this information and synchronize your medical treatment if it is in more than one doctor's hands.

Some drugs have a beneficial effect. Certain antibiotics—troleandomycin (TAO), for example—enhance the effect of steroids, which may make it possible to reduce the steroid dosage. Troleandomycin seems to be most effective with a particular type of steroid, methylprednisolone (Medrol), and can prove very helpful when other attempts to decrease steroids have failed, but it may have unpleasant side effects.

On the other hand, taking steroids with some drugs may not affect the steroids but rather the action of the other drugs. For instance, because steroids tend to make beta-receptors less sensitive, they increase the action of beta-stimulating bronchodilators (albuterol, ephedrine, terbutaline, for example), which may mean an alteration in your maintenance schedule.

A less benign interaction may occur when a diabetic who also has asthma takes steroids for asthma plus the oral hypoglycemic drugs that may be part of the maintenance program for the diabetes. Also, anyone taking diuretics (for a heart condition, for instance), which tend to increase the body's excretion of potassium, may experience a dangerously low potassium level.

You cannot be expected to know or anticipate drug interactions, unless they are based on allergies that you have experienced, but, again, you can help by informing each doctor what drugs other doctors have prescribed and what over-the-counter drugs you may be taking on your own. Do not overlook common OTC drugs like aspirin, which you may have been taking for years and have come to consider harmless; even aspirin can cause harmful side effects if taken in combination with certain prescription drugs. It cannot be emphasized too often that if you have specialists prescribing for you, in addition to your family doctor, be sure they all know everything you are taking.

8

Drugs Recently Introduced

Although many of the drugs used to treat asthma—such as ephedrine—have been known and used for at least five thousand years, there are new or recently developed drugs now available or in the testing stage that show great potential for alleviating and even controlling asthma. Since the cause of asthma is still not known, none offers the promise of a cure, but they do show a much broader understanding of, and interesting new approaches to, this puzzling illness.

European countries have long been in the forefront of much of the new asthma drug development, and many of these drugs come to the United States from abroad, after considerable clinical testing and with wide general use and acceptance behind them. The Federal Drug Administration (FDA) must still apply its own approval process to any new drug, even one that is widely accepted in other counties, and inevitably, this has sometimes delayed the availability of a new and effective drug to our medical community.

Although the FDA has been criticized for its sometimes lengthy approval process, it has recently made exceptions—notably in the case of new AIDS drugs—in order to speed up (and sometimes even circumvent) the approval process in the interests of making a drug available more quickly. On the other hand, if it had not been for the thoroughness of the FDA approval process, the United States would have joined most other countries of the world in approving thalidomide, and an even greater number of tragically deformed babies would have been born.

Although each country has its own approval process, worldwide interest and research in the development of new respiratory drugs helps everyone. The World Health Organization (WHO) oversees and coordinates global drug development and use and annually examines and evaluates clinical results. While no country is bound by WHO's recommendations, the organization disseminates information as to what is happening in other countries and encourages the coordination of research throughout the world.

An interesting development in the drug field has been the increasing number of drugs already approved for other diseases and subsequently found to be of value in treating entirely unrelated diseases, including asthma. Once a drug is approved, a physician is given a great deal of leeway as to how and for what purpose he or she prescribes it. This makes possible an open-minded look at drug reaction patterns. Also, the perception that asthma is in some way caused by an overactive immune system has directed attention to a broader area, away from the focus on the immediate physiological reactions of constricted airways toward a consideration of the immune system as a whole.

A further advance was made possible when the importance of inflammation as an asthma trigger was realized and more aggressive treatment with anti-inflammatory drugs was begun. Steroids, dramatically successful in reducing the inflammation of arthritis, proved equally helpful with severe asthma. Unfortunately, because of the side effects of long-term oral steroid use, such use is now considered a last resort, but short-term courses are widely used to stabilize recurrent acute asthma.

The development of inhaled steroids appears to have overcome most of the side effects, although steroids have not been used as inhalants long enough for American physicians to feel entirely certain of their long-term effect on nasal and throat linings. At present they are being prescribed widely but carefully observed to determine whether their long-term use produces any negative effects.

Asthma drug research is aimed primarily in four directions: to control allergic reactions; to influence immune system reactions; to control, prevent, or reverse bronchospasm; and to prevent or reverse inflammation reactions.

Here is a brief survey of some of the most recently introduced drugs.

Cromolyn Sodium (Intal in the United States, Lomudal in Europe and England)

Cromolyn sodium evolved from work with khellin, a drug obtained from the seeds of an eastern Mediterranean plant, which had been used in folk medicine for centuries as a smooth muscle relaxant (although cromolyn itself is thought to have no smooth muscle relaxant effect). Cromolyn was introduced in Great Britain in January 1968, after years of worldwide clinical testing, and became available in the United States in 1975, where it was unenthusiastically received by much of the medical community. Although it not strictly speaking a new drug introduction, it is only recently that it has begun to come into its own.

The action of cromolyn is different from that of other antiasthmatic medications. Although not yet clearly understood, it does not block the production of mast-cell mediators but appears to block cells from releasing them when it is used before exposure to an allergen. It may prevent mast cells from releasing histamine, for example (which might otherwise trigger asthma symptoms). In addition, it seems in some way to actually reduce twitchy airway reactivity in general. Unlike various other asthma drugs, it is not a bronchodilator, has no apparent anti-inflammatory effect, and does not increase the level of cyclic AMP (cAMP).

Although originally thought to be useful primarily for allergic (extrinsic) asthma (it also relieves rhinitis), cromolyn has been found to work equally well for nonallergic (intrinsic) asthma. As a result, its use is no longer confined primarily to children, and it is thought to have a generally beneficial application regardless of age. It is well regarded by athletes because of its effectiveness in preventing EIA and EIB (exercise-induced asthma and broncho-spasm), but it must be used well in advance of a competitive event (or even better, as an adjunct to a daily maintenance schedule) to give it time to take effect. Since it is not effective after symptoms have started, it is not useful as a bronchodilator in the event of an actual episode.

When treatment with cromolyn is first started, the beneficial effects may take as long as a month to surface, so someone taking it for the first time should not expect instant results but should be patient and give it a fair trial. Since there seem to be practically no side effects caused by even long-term use of cromolyn, it tends to be well tolerated by those who have had a problem with other drugs. It is especially useful, therefore, for patients who cannot tolerate theophylline or adrenergic medications and is often the replacement drug in those instances.

Cromolyn is also very helpful in reducing the need for oral steroids, but they may still be needed for sudden, acute episodes, where cromolyn is inappropriate.

The unpredictable nature of asthma reactions, especially those due to circumstances and trigger exposure beyond your control, makes it particularly important for you to understand how each drug works and to carefully note your doctor's instructions for dealing with these situations as well as for complying with your maintenance program. Since the average asthma regimen usually requires regular or backup use of several drugs, it is fortunate that cromolyn is compatible with most other drugs.

Cromolyn sodium is available as an inhalant in a number of devices, and it should be possible to find one that works for you. It cannot be taken orally, since it is so poorly absorbed in the gastrointestinal tract that it would be difficult to take a large enough dose in tablet form. Do not confuse the capsules that come for insertion in the Spinhaler (see pages 76–77) with oral medication; they are not to be swallowed. If you were to absent-mindedly do so, it would not harm you, but neither would it help your asthma.

Side Effects

As we have indicated, cromolyn sodium has very few side effects, and it is estimated that only 2 percent of users experience any of them. With the powder form the most annoying is a cough, which the newer spray form seems to have eliminated. Other possible but seldom experienced side effects may be dryness of the mouth, throat irritation, and hoarseness. If you are bothered by any of these, you can always discuss it with your doctor. (They may be due to other medications you are taking along with the cromolyn sodium, so be sure to have your list handy.)

How to Use Cromolyn Sodium

Your doctor will determine the specifics of size of dose and frequency of use and explain the place of cromolyn in your regimen. Since its function is preventive, you may be given it on a regular maintenance regimen, along with other drugs. If, however, you are subject to occasional asthma—for instance, only during certain seasons of the year, perhaps when ragweed pollen is airborne in the fall—early pretreatment with cromolyn may be advised, starting before the season begins. Since the start of pollen seasons varies considerably, depending on precipitation, weather, and other influences, be sure to allow enough margin for possible early pollen onset—once the season has started, it will be too late.

In the event that you anticipate a situation where you may be exposed to something that can trigger a bronchospasm—such as going to a smoky restaurant or cocktail party, visiting a friend with a house pet, or exercising outdoors on a cold or windy day—your doctor may suggest that you take cromolyn at least fifteen or twenty minutes before you will be exposed. In addition, a period of exposure that stretches over several hours should be checked with your doctor; he or she may suggest using your inhaler a second time.

If you are subject to late-phase-response asthma, cromolyn can be used to prevent both ordinary asthma (immediate asthma) and the late-phase type. Dr. Gary L. Larsen, associate professor of pediatrics, University of Colorado School of Medicine, writing in "The Pulmonary Late-Phase Response" (*Hospital Practice,* November 15, 1987), comments on the versatility of pretreatment with cromolyn: "Moreover, it is remarkable that both late-phase and immediate pulmonary responses are blocked by cromolyn sodium. The drug may inhibit mediator release from effector cells, such as mast cells and basophils . . . but its value is chiefly prophylactic."

If you forget to pretreat yourself before exposure, it won't help to take cromolyn when you are already having difficulty breathing; you'll need to use a bronchodilator, such as an albuterol inhaler. However, if you have not yet started wheezing, it might be worth trying a puff of cromolyn; it might still help, and it won't hurt.

Ketotifen (Zaditen in Europe and Elsewhere)

Ketotifen is a new synthetic nonsteroidal, anti-inflammatory drug (NSAID) that, like cromolyn sodium, is a preventive rather than a bronchodilator. Long available for asthma (as Zaditen) in Europe, the Far East, and South America, it is expected to be available by prescription in the United States in the near future.

There is nothing that new about NSAIDs; you are familiar with them as aspirin, ibuprofen, and indomethacin, and asthmatics are generally advised to avoid them, since they can sometimes bring on a severe, rapid-onset asthmatic attack in sensitive individuals. It is thought that as many as 20 percent of asthmatics may have an NSAID sensitivity. (See pages 70–71.)

Like cromolyn, ketotifen appears to be quite safe for those

not sensitive to NSAIDs. The only important side effect is drowsiness, which occurs in approximately 15 percent of adult users and even less frequently among children. If drowsiness occurs initially, it tends to wear off after two weeks of use. As with other NSAID drugs, the nature of its action is not completely understood.

Ketotifen may take longer to work than cromolyn (it requires four to twelve weeks of use before it becomes effective), but it can be taken orally, which many users may find more convenient than adding another inhaler, and it can usually be taken only twice a day.

What Ketotifen Does and How It Does It

Like all preventive asthma drugs, the primary function of ketotifen is to prevent asthma rather than to treat asthma flares and active bronchospasm. It appears to work no matter what triggers are causing asthma symptoms but is thought to be particularly effective against allergens, including food. Since the majority of asthma triggers are allergens, this covers a lot of asthmatics. Also, as was the case with cromolyn, it may be that further studies will show that ketotifen actually has a much wider range of effectiveness.

Ketotifen, like cromolyn, is thought to work through its action on calcium, thereby somehow blocking the effect of an allergen on the mast cells. When effective, ketotifen—as does any preventive asthma drug—reduces the need for steroids and bronchodilators. The full extent of its usefulness is yet to be determined.

Calcium Antagonists (Calcium Channel Blockers)

Studies increasingly indicate that calcium plays a major role in the triggering of asthma symptoms. The theory is that calcium must enter the mast cell if the cell is to be able to release histamine and other chemical mediators (which we now believe trigger asthma symptoms). Preventing it from getting into the cell appears to block this chemical release. Calcium is also thought to play a role in bronchospasm and the excess secretion of mucus.

Here again is an instance where a type of drug previously found effective for another disease may be of use in controlling asthma. Calcium antagonists have been shown to help angina pectoris, some arrhythmias, and other cardiac diseases. Now two such drugs, veraparmil and nifedipine, appear to show considerable promise as preventive asthma drugs. Some studies seem to indicate they may have successfully prevented extrinsic asthma and had some beneficial effect on EIA and EIB. Whether or not they prove useful, it is encouraging that so many new directions are being explored.

Nonsteroidal Anti-inflammatory Drugs (NSAIDs)

In spite of their undesirable side effects, steroids continue to be used more and more because of their strong anti-inflammatory action in controlling asthma. Meanwhile ongoing research has strongly focused on the search for a nonsteroidal anti-inflammatory drug that would have the benefits but not the disadvantages of steroids.

As we have seen, not only do many of the nonsteroid anti-inflammatory drugs that already exist appear to have no provable beneficial effect on asthma but some, such as aspirin, can actually be harmful. If you are aspirin-sensitive, it may be best to avoid all NSAIDs, even though many are common over-the-counter drugs widely used for relief of headaches, menstrual cramps, and mild pain. Arthritis is frequently treated with large doses of aspirin in one of its various guises; if you need aspirin and have asthma, be sure to point out to your doctor this juxtaposition (you may be going to one doctor for the arthritis and another for the asthma, so you are the one who must make the connection unless your family doctor is overseeing both specialists).

A rapid-onset, severe attack can occur even when there has been no previous indication of NSAID sensitivity, so it is part of good self-management to learn some of the commonly used OTC products that contain NSAIDs and to act quickly, with appropriate measures as taught by your physician, to counteract any resultant unexpected, sudden, severe attacks. Your doctor may advise calling an ambulance as soon as you have the least reaction to such medication, so as to lose no time in case your measures are inadequate to control the attack.

Ideally, of course, if you have asthma, avoidance of NSAIDs—as with any trigger—is best.

Anticholinergic Drugs

To understand the purpose of anticholinergic drugs, it is necessary to go into a little physiology. The vagus nerve (part of the parasympathetic nervous system) releases the cholinergic mediator acetylcholine (histamine) when stimulated. This chemical can trigger asthma by constricting airway muscles and increasing mucus production. It is thought that acetylcholine can make matters worse by also activating the mast cells to release their constricting mediators. If you've been reading about other asthma drugs, you know that the next inevitable step was for someone to develop a drug that blocks the production of acetylcholine, and that is exactly what happened.

The drug that was developed was atropine, which comes from solanaceous plants (these include deadly nightshade, henbane, and jimsonweed), known at least since 3000 B.C. as magic potions, deadly poisons, and medicines. (In spite of its off-putting name, deadly nightshade is also the source of another old and useful medication still used today, belladonna.)

In the eighteenth century, the British, borrowing from the pharmacology of ancient India, used dried jimsonweed (another atropine-containing plant) to make "asthma cigarettes," and advertisements for them can be found in early newspapers of the American colonies. "Asthma cigarettes" were sold in the United States as late as the 1930s when epinephrine supplanted it as the standard treatment for asthma.

As our medical knowledge increases, we sometimes find ourselves returning to ancient remedies, and in a way, that is what has happened with atropine, which once again is finding its place in asthma medication. As usual, it was first reintroduced in Europe and Canada, and it is only in the last few years that it has received FDA approval and is now available for use with asthma in the United States.

Ipratropium Bromide (Atrovent)

Ipratropium bromide is an atropine derivative. It is available as Atrovent, a bronchodilating inhaler. When compared to sympathomimetic bronchodilators, it is generally slower-acting (fifteen to thirty minutes as against five minutes for albuterol) and slower to peak but lasts twice as long (up to eight hours).

It is almost entirely free of side effects, except for a dry mouth, and is effective against all the usual asthma triggers (including allergic, nonallergic, and exercise-induced asthma), although it is more effective against intrinsic than extrinsic asthma. It seems to work especially well against inhaled intrinsic asthma triggers, such as cigarette smoke, cold air, and industrial irritants. Atrovent comes in oral and injectable forms but is most commonly used for asthma as an inhalant.

Another good feature of ipratropium bromide is that it is compatible with sympathomimetic drugs, such as theophylline, and with steroids, each increasing the effect of the other and allowing the amount of the dosage of the latter drugs to be decreased. As with cromolyn sodium, its effect may be variable and it is not suitable for everyone; it is effective for all ages, although it seems to work especially well for young children and the elderly.

Keeping Track of New Drug Introductions

Some people prefer not to get too involved in the details and to leave the field of drugs to their physicians. That is not inconsistent with self-care so long as you know the generic and brand names of the drugs you are taking, the dosage, when and how you are to take them, possible side effects, and what they are supposed to do for you. Only in that way can you help your physician by reporting whenever you experience untoward side effects or are simply not getting the results you were told to expect.

If, on the other hand, you like to know more about what is being done for asthma, you can keep an eye out for newspaper and magazine articles on the subject. There are also a number of health magazines and some good health letters that keep up with new drugs. One of your best sources is your local pharmacist. Even the pharmacy in a chain store has a trained pharmacist, and if you pick a time when he or she is not busy filling prescriptions and answering the phone, the pharmacist will probably be happy to take a break and talk to you about new asthma medications.

Just don't ask too many questions or take up too much time at any one session, and of course, always leave if other customers arrive. Once the pharmacist gets to know you, you will have a handy, knowledgeable source for anything you want to know about drugs.

9

Treating Asthma
with Inhalers

What Is an Inhaler?

Asthma drugs come in many forms: tablets, liquids, inhalants, injections, and gels. Some, such as intravenous preparations and injections, are suitable only (with some exceptions) for professional medical use. Others may be used by the patient with the doctor's guidance. Among the latter are the medications suitable for inhalation.

There are three kinds of asthma drugs that are available in inhalers and/or inhaling devices. (They may also come in other forms.)

1. Adrenalin and Adrenalin-like medications
2. cromolyn sodium
3. corticosteroids

Since your physician is likely to prescribe one or more of them for your asthma, you will be able to follow his or her instructions more easily and achieve maximum control of your health if you know and understand what they are, how they act, and what they may be expected to do to mitigate symptoms.

The device that creates an inhalable spray to deliver these medications is called an inhaler. There are two inhalation methods used, breath-activated and propellant-activated.

Inhalers for asthma drugs vary from the simple, hand-held type to more complicated tabletop models for home or hospital use, such as nebulizers. Anyone using the more complicated models will be given extensive training in how to use them; this discussion will be confined to hand-held models.

Metered-Dose Inhalers (MDI)

The most common type of inhaler is a metered-dose inhaler, referred to as an MDI, in which a pressurized canister of medication is inserted into a holder. When the canister in this type of MDI is pressed down, a predetermined (metered) and uniform dose of medication is delivered by a propellant gas and comes out as a fine spray or mist. The term "aerosol" is used to describe both this type of canister and the spray or mist dispensed by it.

Other MDI systems deliver the medication by passing a stream of your inhaling air over the drug, which picks it up and ejects it as spray. Since both methods deliver a uniform dose each time the device is activated, you do not have to measure or be in any way responsible for ejecting the correct dose; the amount of medication is totally controlled by the device. What is within your control, however, is the technique needed to get a sufficient amount of the medication into your airways. Although this is not difficult to master, it requires understanding how to do it and a certain amount of concentration until correct procedure becomes a habit.

Cromolyn sodium, if used in powder form, requires a different kind of inhaler, the Spinhaler, which was developed especially for it. The Spinhaler is estimated to deliver 50 percent of the medication to the airways. Instead of relying on the user's timing, the Spinhaler synchronizes the nebulization of the drug with the user's own inhalation, ensuring that an optimum dosage actually reaches the airways, rather than being deposited on the back of the throat (as can happen with improper use of the standard propellant type of inhaler). Now cromolyn sodium also comes in liquid form for those who prefer the standard propellant inhaler.

Ventolin, on the other hand, which up to now has used the standard propellant inhaler, has now come out with a powder form. The inhalers for this include the Rotahaler, now sold in the United States, and the Diskhaler, which is available in Canada and will possibly be available in the United States shortly. For a more detailed discussion of these three devices, see Chapter 21.

(I would not burden you with all these details and terms, but you will find them referred to constantly by physicians and therapists and in books and articles on asthma, and they are sometimes not explained or defined.)

How to Use a Propellant Inhaler

It is generally estimated that with the standard inhaler only about 10 percent of the inhaled drug actually reaches the lungs; the remaining 90 percent is deposited on the lining of the mouth and throat. Since enough of the drug still reaches the airways to achieve the desired effect—such as reversing bronchospasm—this is satisfactory. But getting the 10 percent to the airways is essential, and only proper technique can ensure that it will happen.

Incorrect technique tends to follow a pattern. On planning to use the inhaler, the person shakes it and then puts it in the mouth, as far back as possible, closing the lips over it. He or she then tries to breathe in deeply while pressing down the canister to release the medication. Not surprisingly, the result is often a quick press, followed by a quick inhalation, and a moment's wait to see if relief follows. When relief is not forthcoming immediately, the second puff (two puffs are the usual dose) is likely to be taken too soon. In a situation where breathing has become uncomfortable suddenly, perhaps because of exposure to a trigger such as tobacco smoke, the natural tendency is the same—to grab the inhaler and inhale quickly.

Most doctors agree that only a slow inhalation can get an effective dose as deeply into the lungs as necessary, at the same time leaving a minimum of residue on the mouth and throat. Since the spray usually contains some larger particles (not medication), it would be best to inhale only the medicated spray. Unfortunately, there is no consensus on how to achieve this goal.

One suggestion that has been made is to hold the inhaler a couple of inches or so away from your open mouth (too far for the larger particles to travel and near enough so that the aerosoled spray does not land on the back of the throat but instead is drawn down into the airways), then press down the canister while inhaling deeply. Unfortunately, I find this almost impossible to do—my aim just isn't that good. In practice, the spray usually ends up on the side of my mouth or the tip of my nose. Many doctors teach this method, and I know a number of people who use it successfully. It's worth a try if that's the way you are taught; you may do it successfully without any difficulty.

Another suggestion is to position the inhaler right in front of your open mouth, touching the edge of your lips, and proceed from there.

A foolproof method is to use a simple device called a spacer, which holds the dispersed medication briefly, trapping the large particles and releasing the spray when you inhale. One version of this, the Aerochamber, made by the Monahagan Medical Corporation in Plattsburgh, New York, is a round blue plastic tube with a rubber opening that fits closely around the dispensing end of the inhaler. The other end goes in your mouth and contains a valve, which helps to trap more large particles. To use, you simply insert the mouth of the inhaler into one end of the tube, shake as usual, and then, with the other end of the spacer in or in front of your mouth, press the canister. There are other styles by other manufacturers, and your doctor or respiratory therapist may have a preference.

This type of device is especially good for children because it eliminates the need for perfect synchronization between pressing down on the canister and breathing in. The two actions need not be simultaneous and will work even if you inhale shortly after the medication is expelled from the canister into the device. The time elapsed between pressing down on the canister and breathing in from the spacer should not be more than a few seconds.

Regardless of what you use, the basic technique consists of exhaling as much air as possible, through pursed-lip breathing, then pressing the canister while *slowly* inhaling the medicated spray for five seconds. Do this gently, not trying *too* hard to breathe deeply, or you may cough and spoil the effect. Hold this inhaled breath for ten seconds, then breathe out through your nose.

If the medication is a bronchodilator, wait at least five minutes before the next puff; ten is even better. The waiting gives the bronchodilator time to at least partially open the airways so that the second puff can reach further down into the lungs.

Never take the second puff right after the first without waiting. If the doctor says, for example, "Take two puffs two times a day," he may neglect to mention the waiting time in between, assuming that you already know about it. Without the waiting time the second puff cannot do its job because the airways will not have relaxed, and you will not be getting the medication as far down as you should.

No matter which method is used, always tilt the head upward (with the inhaler upright but pointing slightly down into your mouth) before inhaling. This places the airways in a better position to receive the spray and reduces the likelihood of the spray hitting the back of your throat.

If you fail to get any relief from a bronchodilator after your first puff, consider the possibility that the canister is empty. Take your backup inhaler (presumably full) and heft it in one hand, with the one you are using in the other hand; this comparison of the two weights may help you tell if any medication is left in the current inhaler. If you still can't tell, use the backup for your second puff; there will be a noticeable difference between the effect from a full cartridge and from an empty one.

If by any chance two puffs don't bring relief within five or ten

How to Tell When the Canister Is Empty

Since the canister is completely enclosed, it is sometimes difficult to tell whether all the medication has been used up. A full canister is heavy and easy to recognize, but one that is empty is not, partly because when shaken, it still seems to contain some liquid.

The most obvious thing to do would seem to be to press down and see whether anything comes out. Unfortunately, that is no help at all because the propellant continues to come out after the medication has been used up and the canister is, as far as medication is concerned, empty.

Another possibility might be to mark on the calendar when you start on a fresh canister and count ahead two hundred puffs, according to your maintenance schedule of two or three double puffs or so a day. That doesn't work either, because there are times when you may have been told to use the inhaler—just before exercising, for instance—that are not part of your maintenance schedule.

Another method of determining whether a canister is empty is to drop it into a bowl of water, the idea being that if it floats it's empty. This system works very well, but I noticed recently that the directions for doing this, which used to be found on some manufacturers' product information sheets that come with the canister, are no longer included.

I phoned the manufacturer of the Ventolin inhaler to inquire as to whether this is a good idea. Since the contents are under pressure and have a very good seal, the representative said, it is unlikely that any water could leak in. But no one these days likes to take even the slightest risk of anything untoward happening, so the representative would not recommend the practice.

I then asked what the company did suggest the user do to determine whether the canister was empty. He said that inasmuch as a canister holds about two hundred doses, one could make a written note every time he or she took a puff and stop at two hundred.

I tried this and found it didn't work very well, so now I have gone back to just comparing the canister I am using to a full one and also to one I know is empty (because I tested it with the water method, not planning to use it again), and I can tell by the heft about how full it is.

If you use an inhaler without getting any relief at all, always consider the possibility that it is empty, but remember that other factors may be causing this problem, and do not keep on trying. The most you might do is try once more with a fresh new inhaler.

minutes, go to your backup procedure. If your doctor hasn't told you what to do in this kind of situation, such as taking an additional puff or two or oral medication, call him or her. This is your first indication that your asthma is more severe than you thought, and unless you have had experience with it and know what to do, it may simply get worse.

Whatever else you do, do not continue to use your inhaler when it isn't helping. Using the inhaler too often is likely, under certain circumstances, to cause the very bronchospasm you are trying to avoid.

You cannot be in control of your asthma without advance planning. It is important for you and your doctor to anticipate the kinds of problems that commonly arise and for you to learn what to do at such times.

How to Use the Spinhaler

Since cromolyn sodium (Intal) is now available as a spray, the Spinhaler, used with cromolyn sodium in powder form, may not appeal to you. However, having both forms does provide a choice, so you may as well know about the Spinhaler, which differs from the propellant inhaler.

The medication, in the form of a capsule, is inserted in a cup set in a propellerlike rotor that spins when air is inhaled with the device in the mouth. To insert the capsule, follow the directions that come in the package. Once the capsule is in place and ready to use, the action of the Spinhaler propels (spins) the medication into the inhaled air as you draw it into your airways. Medication is automatically released only when you inhale, so no coordination (between inhaling and releasing the medication) is necessary.

When inhaling, draw your breath in rapidly (rather than slowly as with other inhalers), with the head tilted backward. Then hold it for about ten seconds, and repeat the procedure until all the powder has been inhaled. Just looking at the capsule will tell you whether any powder is still unused.

An excellent instruction sheet accompanies the Spinhaler, showing how to use and care for it. Your doctor will undoubtedly want to check that you are using it correctly and will explain why it is not useful if you are having an acute asthma attack. (NOTE: If you have no problem in synchronizing pressing down the canister and breathing in the medicated spray that is then released—as is required by a regular MDI inhaler—remember that cromolyn sodium (Intal) now comes in spray form, too. And even if you do, a spacer can be used with cromolyn as well as with any other medication suitable for an MDI inhaler. In addition, cromolyn sodium can be used with a portable nebulizer. Depressing an activator button releases the medication as a mist, which can be breathed in from the large mouthpiece.)

Advantages of Inhaled Medications

Inhaled asthma drugs have certain advantages over other forms. First of all, an inhaler is handy; it can be kept in a pocket, attaché case, or handbag and used unobtrusively, even in public. Since there is no way of knowing when you will have trouble breathing or even have an attack, most asthmatics who use an inhaled bronchodilator tend to carry it with them at all times. Many have a backup inhaler, either at home or, if traveling, in luggage. Given the importance of the quick relief an inhaled bronchodilator provides, a backup is a good idea.

Pills require a container, and getting one out of a pillbox attracts attention; also, most people need water to swallow them. Syrups are obviously awkward to take when away from home or office and require a spoon, which must then be washed.

Children can carry an inhaler in a pocket or pencil case, and for added security, a second one can be left with the school nurse, who will, in any case, have been briefed on the student's needs.

Another advantage to an inhaled asthma drug is that it goes directly to the site—the airways—and therefore not only acts more quickly but does so with a smaller dose than would be required orally. Also, because the drug does not get into the bloodstream and travel through the body, many side effects either do not occur or are minimized.

Achieving relief with the least amount of drug in one's body is always desirable; in the case of steroids it is especially important. Not only can the effective inhaled dose usually be smaller than the oral dose but also, because it is not ingested, the worrisome side effects do not occur. If you are taking both oral and inhaled steroids, the inhaled may prove so effective that your doctor will be able to discontinue the oral altogether.

Disadvantages of Inhaled Medications

To some extent, the disadvantages vary with the nature of the drugs taken.

Inhaled Bronchodilators

Inhaled medication may not reach the airways because of obstruction, such as mucus or an extremely tight bronchospasm; the less air that is getting through, the less inhaled medication you get. If the symptoms are not relieved by using the inhaler, an oral medication or an injection is indicated and should be gotten promptly. Be sure your physician advises the procedure to follow if your usual inhaled medication does not seem to be helping as it should. Do not, as we have said, keep using the inhaler when it proves ineffective.

Inhaled Steroids

The same problem discussed above applies to inhaled steroids and to any other inhaled medication, but steroids also have certain unique disadvantages. The one that occurs most frequently, thrush, is a fungus infection that shows up as white patches on mucous membranes, especially in the mouth and back of the throat. Since it doesn't cause any discomfort, when using inhaled steroids, make a point of routinely examining your mouth (lifting up your tongue) and the back of your throat.

Thrush is usually easily prevented by thoroughly rinsing the mouth and gargling the throat immediately after using the inhaler. If you also use a nasal steroid, taking the mouth and nasal steroid inhalations one after the other, rinse and gargle for both drugs at one time.

Occasionally, inhaled nasal steroids cause slight bleeding, which is noticeable when you blow your nose. Another side effect is hoarseness, which may gradually get worse.

Always notify your doctor if you think you have any of these side effects; he or she may want to temporarily reduce the steroid or prescribe a special medicated gargle to clear it up. Your doctor may also recommend nasal lavage.

Inhaled Cromolyn Sodium

Cromolyn sodium does not work as an oral medication, so it is available only as an inhalant, but it comes in three different inhalant types; the Spinhaler, an MDI aerosol, and a nebulizer. In addition to its tendency to cause throat irritation or dryness, as we have already mentioned, the powder form may make you cough. This is easily overcome by switching to the new metered-dose inhaler for nasal inhalation, which eliminates the cough reaction. If you are having a problem with the powder form (using the Spinhaler), ask your doctor if you could switch to one of the other forms and inhalant devices. The drug itself is the same no matter how it is delivered.

Another disadvantage to the Spinhaler is having to unwrap the capsule and insert it in the cup, which is more time-consuming than just reaching for the inhaler. However, since cromolyn sodium is a preventive medication, not indicated in an acute asthma situation, the little extra time involved is not critical. Also, now that it is available as a metered-dose inhaler, it is just as easy to use as your other inhalers.

Having two different medications as inhalers should not be confusing, because usually the colors are quite different even if the design is similar.

Part Three

What You Can Do

10

How to Work with Your Doctor

Most of the time you will be alone with your asthma, and how you manage then is in your hands. But an important part of managing successfully is working well with your doctor.

The Doctor-Patient Relationship

Like any relationship, the one between doctor and patient should be a two-way street, with mutual respect and communication. The patient needs to understand the whys and wherefores of treatment, know what to expect from medication, and feel free to ask about an article that describes a new, possibly helpful drug without the doctor taking offense or feeling the patient is trespassing. The doctor, in turn, should have an open mind about a patient's reports of atypical drug reactions, new symptoms, and general progress, allow time to explain changes in regimes and to reassure an anxious patient, and feel that the patient has confidence in his expertise and is not hostile.

Most doctors no longer attempt to remain aloof from the patient or expect whatever they say to be accepted unquestioningly, but some do get irritated and touchy when patients try to discuss medical aspects of their problem. With the greater degree of sophistication and knowledge of today's patients, an authoritative attitude doesn't sit too well, and the patient may then have a conflict—whether to look for a new doctor or to put up with this condescending attitude because the physician, in spite of being difficult to work with, is competent.

At a recent breathing club meeting the speaker was from the hospital's pharmacy department. He discussed in considerable detail the most commonly prescribed asthma medications and encouraged the audience to interrupt whenever they had a question. About half an hour into his talk the questions became so numerous that he scrapped the rest of his outline and settled down to responding to them. I was surprised and impressed by the audience's knowledge. They included men and women of all ages, with various pulmonary diseases of varying degrees of severity. What they all had in common was a desire to know even more than they already did, to understand as much as possible about their disease and its treatment, and to find out what they could do to improve it or make it easier to live with.

After the talk was over, I went up to the speaker and asked whether he had been surprised by how much the audience knew and how intelligent their questions were. He said no—he found people with asthma and chronic obstructive pulmonary disease knew a great deal about their disease and how to manage it and were always eager to learn more.

It seemed to me that they were bursting with questions they had not been able to ask their doctors, even though most of them had doctors I knew were excellent and fairly forthcoming. The problem, of course, is that even a good and communicative doctor does not have enough time to sit down and talk at length with a patient. Appointments are routinely set fifteen minutes apart, and doctors, who start early in the morning with hospital visits, often skip lunch in order to deal with emergencies. There just isn't much give in the schedule, and this is unfortunate.

If you call with a question, it is often the nurse who conveys question and answer—so the question had better be short and explicit.

I sometimes think the system my children's pediatrician had was a good one: he set aside a time very early in the morning when mothers could call with questions. It wasn't usually necessary to talk at any length, but I always felt I could if I needed to. There were no intermediaries; you dialed the number and the doctor picked up the phone. For a new mother it was total access and total reassurance; for an experienced one it was efficient and completely satisfactory. We tried to be quick so as many mothers as possible could get through, but he never rushed us.

Whether that system would work with an adult practice, I don't know. And perhaps it is heresy to suggest that it might help if doctors determined the number of patients they can handle on the basis of quality, rather than quantity, of care. The standard fifteen-minute office visit, further reduced by interruptions for emergency phone calls and the time the patient takes dressing and undressing in the examination room, just doesn't leave much time for discussion or questions.

Fewer patients would result in a lower income, but presumably those who go into the medical profession do not do so solely for the money. While medicine has become one of the highest-paying professions, it also requires a long and arduous apprenticeship, often graduating with a high burden of debt, and, in private practice, the expense of setting up an office. Potentially, becoming a lawyer or a stockbroker can be a quicker and far less time-consuming route to a comfortable income.

Traditionally, people were attracted to the medical profession because they wanted to help others, and the hardships and, in those days, small recompense were worth the sacrifices because of the personal satisfaction the job brought. The doctor-patient relationship was usually a warm one, and even though doctors actually knew much less and had far less technology at their command, they were perceived as being able to help in most instances and were not personally blamed when things went against them.

These days, it almost seems as if doctoring is all tests and machinery, and the relationship the patient has with the doctor is sometimes less than the relationship with the doctor's business staff. Third-party payment, with health insurance taking care of the bills, creates a further gap, making the relationship even more impersonal and creating an ocean of paperwork that is in itself a source of expense and irritation.

Medicare patients, perceived by some doctors as freeloaders unless they are indigent, are often at a disadvantage because so many of the essential services are not covered; the conscientious doctor who believes in preventive medicine or in the value of spending time talking with the patient for a more thorough diagnosis must do so out of his own pocket, or sends bills the patient is liable for and often cannot pay except with money set aside for medications, food, and shelter.

The doctor-patient relationship is thus jeopardized by the nature of modern medicine, which pushes doctors to a long, rushed, and stressful working day; surrounds them with an ever-growing fund of medical information (but with little time to absorb it), which the media make available more or less accurately to anyone who reads a newspaper or watches TV; and offers expensive tests and treatments, which fear of a malpractice suit may lead doctors to prescribe even though they may not think them strictly indicated.

At a time when successful human relationships seem to be difficult to achieve, at least judging from the high divorce rate, the apparent frequency of child abuse, and other deep societal ills, it is no wonder that the doctor-patient relationship is often unsatisfactory. But it is too important to our well-being to give up on, and we have to do our part to make it work.

The Doctor as a Human Being

When you're not feeling well, it is comforting to think that the doctor will fix everything. You really know, of course, that he—or she—is only human and is limited in how much he can accomplish by the state of medical knowledge and his own expertise. What you may not consider is that he is also limited by being human; he gets tired, he has personal problems, he even gets sick just as you do. Also, he has other patients, some of whom may be sicker than you are and require more of his time and attention.

If most of the time he is accessible and reasonably communicative, an occasional lapse (or even a period when he seems preoccupied) is understandable. Doctors, like soldiers, can call on tremendous resources under special stress, but it is not reasonable to expect them to operate on this level twenty-four hours a day, seven days a week. In choosing a doctor, look at how he is *usually.* If he is usually irritable, uncommunicative, and looking at his watch ten minutes into your fifteen-minute office visit, reevaluate the quality of care he can give you.

As we have discussed, when you have a chronic disease like asthma, you may have more than one doctor. Often your family doctor or internist treats you initially, but he or she may be more knowledgable about gastroenterology or some other area than about asthma and may refer you to a pulmonary specialist (who may also be an internist). Should your problem then be diagnosed as primarily due to allergy, you may next find yourself also in the hands of an allergist. Although each of these doctors is important to you, the greater the specialization, the more liable you are to find the care you receive limited in scope.

Your primary care physician is the first one on the list, and your overall condition is his or her responsibility. Your relationship with this physician is the most critical; usually he or she is the one you call first and the one who coordinates the information generated by any other doctors you see. With asthma and other chronic diseases, you may have an ongoing relationship with the specialists we have mentioned, but with most specialists and with all surgeons your relationship is usually short-term; how you feel about them and get along with them, providing you think them competent, is not quite so important. If, however, your asthma requires fairly regular contact with the specialist, the nature and quality of the relationship is just as important as with your family doctor.

Doctors are themselves ambivalent about how they want to be perceived. On the one hand, they would like to have your confidence and acceptance; on the other hand, they sometimes say, "I'm not God," when a patient or relative looks to them for a miracle and is upset when it is not forthcoming. It is up to you to be realistic and to maintain a happy medium. Avoid making a snap judgment, and unless you have reason to know or feel strongly that the treatment is inappropriate, give it a fair try.

How Doctors Handle Billing

The first impression of a doctor comes when you walk in the door. The physical surroundings are usually pleasant enough, but it is the staff and the little notices and signs that set the tone of the office. A Gallup study done in 1989 for the American Medical Association found that 67 percent of the respondents felt that doctors are too interested in making money, and this feeling is reinforced by the reception area as well as by the billing staff. Most doctors' offices prominently display signs asking you to pay then and there for the services just rendered. And often the person at the window you must pass to exit calls out to you if you try to leave without taking care of your bill.

Although doctors appear to be surprised and hurt by the frequently voiced perception that they are too concerned with the financial side of their practice, they reinforce it by what they do when it comes to paying for medical care. A real-life example is what happened to a woman I know who had just had a colonoscopy. The doctor informed her that she had polyps, which he thought were probably malignant. She took the news fairly well, and they discussed what should be done next. As she put on her coat and prepared to leave, he asked her to pay for the examination at the desk. The bill was $900.

A doctor who would require immediate payment from a patient who has just discovered she probably has cancer should not expect to be considered among the most compassionate and caring of individuals; yet, though this may be an extreme example, it actually happens every day in doctors' offices throughout the land. Patients are usually nervous to begin with when going to a doctor; proof of this is the fact that blood pressure readings are often higher when taken by the doctor than when monitored away from the office or even when taken by the nurse. In addition, a patient may be further unsettled by what the doctor finds.

Under such circumstances, to add the stress of a request for payment on the spot is hardly therapeutic.

Most of the time, in spite of the notices, it is possible to leave without immediate payment. If so, when the bill comes in the mail and the amount is large, it may be necessary to pay in installments. At this point the business aspect of medical care becomes even more evident; more and more doctors' bills charge interest on the unpaid balance. In talking with patients, I have found that many consider this "outrageous," and react with resentment toward the doctor. As the Gallup study revealed, 26 percent of the patients who reported that they respected doctors less than they used to said it was because "they are in it for the money."

What You Can Do to Get Quality Care

What you surely cannot do is be without a doctor. Take something as simple as your present medication regime.

Most of the medications you need are available only by prescription. Even supposing your present medications are controlling your asthma satisfactorily and all you need from the pharmacist are refills, he has to check with the doctor before providing them. Since asthma is not a static condition, your medication needs may change. Ideally, symptoms will occur less frequently and be less severe; conversely, they may worsen. In either case your medications occasionally will need adjusting.

In addition, you may want to ask about a new medication that the FDA has just approved, or you may feel you need a course of cortisone due to an inadvertent exposure to a trigger that has caused a reaction. You may think you know what to do, but without a doctor you won't be able to do it. And no matter how much you think you know, you still do not have a doctor's background, training, and knowledge. Taking control of your asthma won't be successful unless you know your limitations and are wise enough to get a doctor's expert advice and help when you need it.

Compared to a doctor, who must wait for patients to come to him, you are a free agent. You can go to practically any doctor you choose, and it's up to you to find one you think is competent, and whom you can trust and work with. Put at least as much thought and time into finding a family doctor as you do into buying a house or a car or making any other major decision.

Get referrals from friends, but remember to ask about things that matter to you; your friends may have different criteria. You may not require the same degree of hand-holding as one friend and may want to know more about your disease than another. It's not enough to know that your friend likes a doctor; what is important is what about him or her is so great. If you check out a name and get some negative responses, find out what they are based on. Some people would rather not be told all about their illness; they feel that that is the doctor's job and he or she should get on with it without making them uncomfortable.

A primary doctor and a patient have to be a moderately good match, temperamentally and psychologically, if they are to work well together. This isn't always evident on the initial visit; it may take time for a good relationship to develop. But at least try to determine why he is a doctor; there are some doctors who care about their patients and about medicine and some who are more interested in *Medical Economics* and think of what they do as if it were just any job.

There are many different kinds of practices—for instance, private practices, group practices, and HMOs (health maintenance organizations)—and they can affect how you are treated as a patient. A doctor in his or her own private practice is always the one treating you (except for days off or on vacation, when someone else is on call). A doctor in a group practice may be freer to take time off, at which point you may discover that you are not happy with some of the others in the group, and if your doctor is getting older and taking more time off, this could become a real problem. An HMO is entirely different in that you have no say about which doctor you are assigned or even which specialist. Theoretically, you can ask for a change if you really don't like the one you are assigned, but you are still limited to the doctors on the staff and may hesitate to ask for a different doctor because you do not want to be tagged as a "difficult" patient. (That kind of tag goes in your medical record; from then on everyone, from other doctors to insurance companies, will see it. Medical records, like credit records, contain many misjudgments of this sort, but unlike credit records, you have no recourse and cannot have them corrected.)

People tend to be more dependent on doctors than on other types of providers and often keep going to one with whom they are really very dissatisfied. If this has been your situation for any length of time, consider a change. On the other hand, perhaps part of the problem lies with you and can be corrected. (See "Making the Most of an Office Visit" on pages 104–105.)

Some doctors are not good with older people. If your relationship has been a long-standing one, you may now be in a category your doctor does not understand or have empathy with. Caring for older people can be frustrating because they tend to have more chronic illnesses and there is much less a doctor can do to really "cure." Older people also react differently to drugs and treatments; if your doctor has not kept up with new developments in this area, he may not be aware of these differences. It is always a wrench to change a doctor you have a long-term relationship with, but sometimes it is best.

Don't Leave Everything to the Doctor

Doctors are not mind readers. When a doctor asks how you are feeling, he is not just being polite; your input is an important part of his ability to do his best for you. Learn to report all pertinent information as briefly but clearly as possible. Do not edit; a symptom or change in your condition that seems minor to you may be a very important clue.

Try to put yourself in perspective by standing off and looking at your activities, your limitations, and your physical condition so that you can describe them accurately. It's sometimes easy to get used to not feeling well, and to accept ill health as normal. Chances are your asthma can be much better than it is, once your doctor understands your condition and teaches you how to take care of yourself. But he won't be able to help as much as he could, if you tell him you're feeling fine when you're really not.

If you're afraid of sounding as if you're complaining, use that perspective I just mentioned to keep your information factual; maybe think of it as a conversation between two doctors—a consultation, so to speak. It may take practice, but it will help you to maintain a positive outlook and to focus on doing whatever is necessary to get control of your asthma.

11

Compliance— Being a Team Player

In the previous section we saw what the doctor can do for us; now let us see what we can do for ourselves.

Common sense tells us there is little point spending time and money getting a doctor's advice and buying the medication he prescribes if we are not going to take either one, yet often that is what many of us do. I am not speaking of the times when you may think the advice is totally off target, as when a doctor who clearly doesn't have a clue as to what is wrong says, "It's all in your mind—you should get counseling" or "There's nothing wrong with you. Stop focusing on how you feel; get out more and have some fun." A doctor who sometimes says simply, "I don't know what's wrong, but let's give this a try," is a pearl beyond price.

Doctors excuse themselves for coming up with a diagnosis even when they don't have one by saying that patients insist on going away with something concrete, preferably a prescription. "Saying 'I don't know exactly what's wrong with you,' " one doctor told me, "loses the patient's confidence—and very often means that patient will go to another doctor." There is certainly truth in this, and we all know the feeling of relief when we leave the doctor's office with a specific diagnosis, a prescription, and instructions to call in two weeks to report, presumably, how much better we are feeling.

The fact is, we don't always have something wrong with us that needs medical care. Life today is full of stress—at work, at home, from family, friends, fellow workers, strangers, and even ourselves when we feel we have failed to reach goals or messed up a relationship we cared about. Stress can cause physical symptoms, such as headaches and stomach upsets, that can masquerade as disease; many common symptoms can be caused by stress alone. We all need to lighten up and not "make ourselves sick" by letting stress get to us.

On the other hand, a headache may be a symptom of a physical condition that will respond to medical intervention. Since any given symptom has a number of possible causes, the doctor has to be a good enough detective to determine which one is causing your headache; a brain tumor, an allergy, money worries, a fight with your best friend, or stuffed sinuses are just a few of the possibilities he or she has to consider.

If, after questions and an examination, the diagnosis is that nothing is seriously wrong, chances these days are you will not go away with the magic prescription in hand. You may instead be given advice, which is generally not nearly so satisfactory. "Take two aspirin and call me in the morning" has become a joke, but it often does clear up minor problems.

In an effort to distinguish between symptoms with physical causes and stress-related symptoms, a wise doctor long ago invented the placebo. A placebo is a harmless pill the dictionary describes as "a medication prescribed more for the mental relief of the patient than for its actual effect on his disorder." The fact that it often works and actually provides relief is further evidence of the strength of the mind/body connection. The more we learn about the effect our mind has on our body, the less we are surprised that a placebo may alleviate, and sometimes even cure, an actual physical medical problem. If you discover that your doctor has given you a placebo, do not be insulted. His diagnosis may have been accurate: just thinking you were going to feel better may have been all the medicine you needed even though your illness is viral, bacterial, or due to a diseased organ. (The effect a patient's attitude and expectations can sometimes have on overcoming illness is now well known among health care professionals. Norman Cousins has shown by his own experience, described in detail in his best-selling books, that a positive attitude can play a helpful role in recovering even from very serious illness. This is now so widely accepted by the medical profession that Mr. Cousins gives courses in his theories to physicians at a leading medical school (see pages 154–56). A strong will to live can sometimes make the difference between life and death. Today surgeons and operating room nurses are taught not to say negative things during an operation about the patient's chances of recovery so as not to risk affecting that will subconsciously even when the patient is under anesthesia. Newspaper reports of crisis situations, with a patient in intensive care, often quote the surgeon as saying, "She has a chance of making it because she has such a strong will to live.")

It is important not to press anxiously for a prescription or a diagnosis but instead to hope for the best and give the doctor time to determine whether anything is wrong. This may mean tests, further examinations, a referral to a specialist, or simply, "Let's see what develops in the next few days." Try to wait without worrying. Meanwhile you have a decision to make.

Your role at this point is to decide what to do next. If you have confidence in your doctor, you should trust his or her expertise. If you don't, even good advice may not work, and you may need to see another doctor. Trust should not, however, mean totally relinquishing your critical judgment. Try to evaluate your doctor as you would any expert, such as a TV repairman or an auto mechanic. If you have any doubts, there is an easy, nonconfrontational way to check his diagnosis. Today there is always the option of a second opinion, which doesn't involve breaking off with your first physician or hurting his feelings. You can always say your insurance requires it.

Making Compliance Easier

1. *Watch for side effects.* If medication has unpleasant side effects, such as nausea, jitteriness, indigestion, gastric reflux, or insomnia, you may resist taking it. A person already uncomfortable with asthma may not consciously make the connection between these new symptoms and new medication but may unconsciously be turned off to taking the drug. Try to notice, and tell your doctor if you suspect you are experiencing side effects. He or she will be able to help you, either by decreasing the dose or by changing the medication.

Most of the time there will be no side effects, so do not expect them; just be observant.

2. *Have a strategy to help you remember.* It's normal and inevitable to forget sometimes to take medication on schedule. Plan ahead to make it easier to remember, and do not change the schedule without checking with your doctor.

3. *Do not discontinue medication on your own.* Even if you think that you understand the purpose of the medication and that you can tell when to discontinue it, or if you feel really good and decide you don't need it anymore, don't stop without telling the doctor. You may not be quite as knowledgeable as you think you are, and you may also not be aware of certain special factors. For instance, oral steroids (like prednisone) must be discontinued very slowly, and can lead to serious consequences if stopped abruptly. On the other hand, a very short, intense course of steroids follows different rules.

4. *Make taking medication a habit.* Chances are you will be on a regime for some time, long enough to turn it into a habit. Habit forming is a useful device for getting things done without having to think about them; use it to help you comply.

5. *Work lifestyle changes into your daily routine.* If part of getting more exercise means riding an exercise bike every day, build it into your schedule. Try getting up half an hour earlier and riding your bike immediately. Then shower, dress, and breakfast in your usual order. Soon you will fall out of bed and onto the bike without even thinking about whether you feel like it. Of course, if you are having extra trouble with your asthma, or you are especially tired, you may make a conscious decision to skip exercise that day or to do much less. The important thing is not having to decide each time; make it automatic. And always warm up and cool down no matter how short a time you exercise.

6. *Motivate yourself.* You are doing all this because you want to feel better and improve the quality of your life. You want to follow the doctor's orders because you choose to do so, not because he or she is telling you to. Don't hesitate to give yourself an occasional pep talk, and to pat yourself on the back when you've done an especially good job and are feeling particularly well or have handled a crisis promptly and efficiently.

7. *Keep learning.* Every time you take a new medication or try a new exercise or new relaxation technique, learn all you can about it. It will make your asthma more interesting and less emotional. It will also improve your ability to take care of yourself. To comply intelligently, you need to know what to expect and how to evaluate whether it is working.

8. *Don't be a passive patient.* Be a team player, doing your part to make the whole project work. Take responsibility for your area and actively help your doctor help you. The benefit is all yours. If your doctor isn't comfortable with this kind of relationship, you may want to consider changing doctors.

Always give the doctor a chance to explain anything you do not understand about the way he is proceeding. If you have heard of medications or medical procedures that you think might be helpful, try to bring them up in a tactful way. Chances are he has good reasons for his decisions, and he may want to proceed cautiously because your symptoms are ambiguous, indicating several very different possibilities. Sometimes waiting a little for further symptoms to develop, or for current ones to resolve, will save you from going through a number of tests that later turn out to have been unnecessary.

Let us assume, however, that you are diagnosed as having asthma, that you accept the diagnosis, and that a regimen of medication is established. Here is where compliance comes in.

Taking Your Medicine

Compliance, in this instance, basically means taking your medicine exactly and as often as prescribed. In addition, if you want to practice self-care, it means keeping records (as with a peak-flow meter), observing your condition (better, worse), and checking in on schedule with a brief but specific report (what worked and what didn't). Almost every doctor I spoke with said the single most serious difficulty encountered in treating patients was their failure to take medication. Medical journals are full of articles both complaining about this and offering suggestions for dealing with it.

We have all missed taking a pill now and then; sometimes instead of four a day we find at bedtime that we have ended up taking only three. This is such a common occurrence that many home medical advice books tell what to do in that case. It depends on which drug is involved. With some drugs you simply go back on schedule the next day; with others you have to make up the missing medication and perhaps need to check with the doctor as to exactly how to do this. He or she knows it can happen and will appreciate your checking. Write down the instructions you are given in your personal medical record; even with the best intentions you will probably do it again.

The doses of some asthma drugs, such as theophylline, have to be customized for each individual, taking into account the metabolism rate and personal habits (smoking, for instance) so as to achieve and maintain an effective blood serum level. Since the rate at which theophylline is metabolized varies from person to person (see Chapter 6), and since, once the effective level has been established, it must be maintained if your asthma is to be properly controlled, adhering to your medication schedule is especially important.

When you've gone off schedule, you may be tempted to double up your next dose, but with theophylline and a number of other drugs this is not a good idea unless your doctor advises it.

If lack of compliance is due to denial on your part that you are sick and need regular medication, that is a problem you must come to terms with. Asthma is not going to get better if you need medicine and don't take it. In addition, you will make it impossible to get proper medical treatment because the doctor will assume you are following instructions, and if the results are not what he is looking for, he will conclude the medication isn't working for you and may increase or even change it.

Asthma, like many chronic diseases, may require a daily schedule of many different drugs—for instance, the use of a bronchodilating inhaler three or four times a day, along with a steroid inhaler (or maybe even two, if a nasal steroid is included) twice a day. In addition, theophylline, terbutaline, and other medications may need to be taken three times daily. If your asthma suddenly flares, you may need to add, briefly, a somewhat complicated regimen of oral steroid tablets. And if you have hay fever, Seldane or some other antihistamine may be added on a twice-daily basis during the pollen season. Keeping track of all this is quite frankly a bother, and you need to be strongly motivated or you are bound to go off schedule.

The solution is to devise a moderately "forget-proof" system, one that fits in with your regular daily activities. For instance, tablets that may be taken with food can be kept handy in the kitchen where they will be noticed at mealtimes. Since they can usually be distinguished by color, shape, or size, a supply can be carried in a small pillbox or other container when you are at work or having a meal out.

There are a number of inexpensive partitioned containers—usually with seven compartments, one for each day of the week—in various shapes and sizes, that fit handily in a pocket, purse, or briefcase. They can be found in most drugstores and tell you at a glance whether you have taken your day's supply.

If most of the time you are taking medication either at home or at the office, you can clue yourself by the position of the containers (such as standing upright, lying on the side, or placed upside down). This sounds tricky, but it works for me.

Inhalers aren't as critical. If you need them regularly, you won't leave home without one. And generally, it's not quite as serious if you get off schedule. If you forget to use one on

Making the Most of an Office Visit

An office visit to your doctor calls for planning on your part if it is to be successful. Here are some of the things you should do.

1. *Make a list.* As you think of questions (since the last visit or phone call), write them down. Before the visit pull them all together. Almost everyone gets a little nervous in the doctor's office—especially if the doctor seems a bit busy or rushed—and routinely forgets to ask things they meant to. This is the only way to remember.

Many doctors will take the list and read it through themselves to save time, so write it neatly and legibly as if someone else is going to read it.

2. *If you don't understand what is wrong with you, ask for an explanation.* Doctors try to use layman's language but don't always succeed. You can't manage your asthma if you don't understand what is going on; always ask. If the doctor says, "I'm not sure—we'll have to do some tests," I would want to know what tests, but don't ask for more than you want to know.

3. *Write down instructions.* Bring a spiral-bound notebook with firm backing, in case you have to write in your lap, and a ballpoint pen that works. If the doctor tells you to take a two-mile walk three times a week, *write it down.* If he or she changes your medication schedule, write down the new one. Don't count on remembering. The book will also come in handy as a record if you need to see another doctor.

4. *Write down any new prescriptions.* Include the name of the drug, the strength, and when and how often you are to take it. This is not only handy for you, it helps you check the label the pharmacist puts on the prescription bottle. If there is a discrepancy between what you wrote down and what the bottle says, ask the pharmacist about it. If you still are not sure, call the doctor (the nurse can check with him or her for you). Pharmacists don't make mistakes in medications anywhere near as often as hospitals do, but you should exert quality control whenever you can.

5. *Ask about drug interactions.* Also ask the pharmacist, when the prescription is filled.

6. *Ask if there are any food restrictions.* Also ask the pharmacist. Doctors often forget to tell you. Pharmacists often put this information right on the label, but sometimes there isn't that much room. It can make a difference in the effectiveness of the drug.

7. *If you keep a chart of your peak-flow meter readings, bring it with you.* It's often a better indicator of your condition than your personal observation.

8. *If you haven't been feeling well, and you have had a particularly stressful occurrence recently, tell the doctor.* Since stress exacerbates asthma, he or she needs to know if that may be why you are suddenly having increased symptoms.

9. *If you are going to have trouble paying the bill and need to pay in installments, this is the time to talk about it.* The doctor is more likely than the billing clerk to be reasonable. Most (but not all) doctors when directly confronted with a financial situation are willing to work something out with you.

10. *If you are on Medicare and want him to accept the assignment, ask.* Doctors are not going to volunteer to do this, but many will when asked or can be cajoled into it if reluctant. You may have to push a little, but do not hesitate to say if it will be a hardship otherwise.

schedule, you can probably do it when you start noticing that you need it.

Giving Up Smoking

If you are a smoker and have asthma, you will have to give up smoking. It's absolutely essential—no ifs, buts, or maybes. You will also need to avoid, as much as possible, inhaling the smoke from other people's cigarettes; fortunately, this is becoming easier with smoking now banned in so many public places.

Having to give up smoking because you have asthma is a double whammy: not only do you have a stressful illness but now you are denied one of the mechanisms you use to cope with stress.

Addiction to nicotine is very real, very physical, and very difficult to overcome. It is only human to rationalize in an effort to continue smoking, but switching to low-tar cigarettes, smoking fewer a day, or telling yourself the damage is already done so you may as well continue will not improve your asthma.

The best method for breaking the habit depends on the individual. There are many helpful strategies, and your doctor, especially if he or she knows you fairly well, may be able to suggest which one may work for you. Quitting all at once, "cold turkey," seems to be the most effective and quickest method, providing you can do it and providing you realize that it may not work the first time. It is important not to be discouraged and to persist. Each time you will tend to make a little progress until eventually, perhaps after several relapses, you will find you are no longer automatically reaching for a cigarette and finally, best of all, no longer craving one.

There are a number of things you can do to help stop on your own (usually the most successful method), including short-term use of nicotine gum, self-hypnosis, not keeping cigarettes around (bumming them doesn't work so well anymore, since many of your friends will give you a lecture instead of a cigarette), and avoiding friends and acquaintances who still smoke.

Smokers usually smoke under certain circumstances: after a meal, during a coffee break, to "relax" when under stress, automatically when working or on the phone, or if feeling lonely or depressed. The automatic element makes breaking the habit harder; finding a cigarette in your mouth when you don't even remember lighting it, or lighting one and finding a half-finished one still burning in the ashtray, shows how much you need to concentrate to break the pattern.

Try to replace the cigarette with something else. If you are in the habit of smoking after a meal, notice how much longer the pleasure of the meal lingers when the taste of food remains in your mouth instead. End with something you especially like—a good cheese, chocolate sauce on your ice cream—so that you can savor it a bit longer instead of replacing it with the harsh, dry taste of tobacco. If you are stressed or restless, engage in physical activity—a short walk or even a chore like cleaning out a drawer, or a few minutes of calisthenics. Sometimes your fingers almost seem to crave a cigarette; find something else to occupy them, like worry beads, a smooth small stone (the Chinese have many such soothing devices), anything with which you can fiddle, especially if you can concentrate on the pleasure of the way it feels and the smoothness of its texture.

More people are giving up smoking today than ever before, and more ways to do it have been developed. Don't hesitate to talk about your problem, and you'll find most people sympathetic and helpful.

It shouldn't be too hard to get motivated when we now know how harmful smoking is even for a healthy person. You'll add years to your life, decrease your risk of heart disease, lung cancer, and emphysema. Your food will taste better, your stamina will increase, your clothes and hair won't smell of stale cigarette smoke, and, at today's prices, you'll save a bundle; start a piggy bank with your daily savings and earmark the money for little luxuries you wouldn't normally indulge in.

12

Recognizing and Dealing with Asthma Triggers

What Are Triggers?

Webster's defines a trigger as "a stimulus that initiates a physiological or pathological process" and gives as an example: "the sight or odor of food may be a trigger for salivation." In other words, food makes your mouth water. An asthma trigger is anything that acts as a stimulus to initiate the symptoms (process) of asthma, which can include bronchial constriction, increased mucus secretion, and difficulty breathing.

Asthma triggers may be either inhaled, eaten, touched, or injected, but regardless of the way they are introduced into the body, the reaction will be the same if you have asthma and if that particular substance is a trigger for your asthma.

We still do not know the underlying reason for the adverse immune system reactions that characterize asthma, but centuries of careful observation have established that almost anything in the environment can set off an asthmatic reaction if you have

Is Asthma a Psychosomatic Disease?

For many years it was thought that asthma was not just a physical but also partly a psychologically induced disease. Profiles were drawn of the "typical" asthmatic, one who was nervous, high-strung, a bit of a hypochondriac, and not especially stable emotionally. Many years ago before I got asthma, a gynecologist once told me that it was fortunate it was my husband, not I, who had asthma, since asthmatics were not ideally suited emotionally, "because of their nerves," to be mothers.

It is only comparatively recently that the relationship between asthma and the emotions has come to be better understood. New studies of the mind/body connection have shown that asthma is not caused by psychological factors, but they can exacerbate it. Anxiety, stress, fearfulness, which can all bring on asthma symptoms, will not do so unless the disease already exists. Since asthma is the result of an overactive immune system, it is obvious that these factors, all of which lower the immune system, are liable to cause an asthmatic response, and that is what sometimes does occur.

Unfortunately, not everyone is aware that asthma is no longer considered a psychosomatic ailment; it is even possible to encounter a physician who still believes it is. Examples commonly used to bolster this viewpoint include the case of the asthmatic woman who was allergic to roses and had an asthma flare upon being confronted with a lifelike artificial rose. With increased knowledge of the mind/body relationship, we now know that such a reaction is not inconsistent with the fact that asthma is not caused by psychological factors; the anxiety occasioned by the thought of exposure to a strong allergen (in this case, a rose) may indeed bring on an asthmatic attack but, again, not unless the disease is already present in the patient. Fear alone is a potent trigger.

Most people with a chronic disease tend to acquire certain specific fears associated with the disabilities caused by their disease. For example, a person with an inner ear difficulty, which affects balance, may be afraid of falling—but the fear of falling has not caused the disease.

When you realize that embarrassment can make you blush (a physical reaction) or fear cause a loss of bladder control (clearly a physical reaction), it is no wonder that in asthmatics certain emotional situations can bring on an attack. It is helpful for the asthmatic to understand this because stress can sometimes be anticipated, possibly controlled, or at least considerably reduced by stress management and relaxation techniques. (This is discussed in detail in Chapter 14.) Once you have mastered these techniques, you will find yourself better able to prevent mild asthma from developing to a more severe stage. At the very least you will not feel so helpless and afraid, and you will be better able to evaluate the seriousness of your symptoms.

asthma and if you are already allergic to it or have developed a sensitivity to it. It needs to be emphasized that many asthma triggers are intrinsically harmless substances that are potentially harmful only to asthmatics.

It is generally accepted that you cannot be sensitive to something to which you have not been exposed, so usually what trigger your asthma are substances common to your everyday environment: foods, animals, plants, insects, clothing, weather, and even the air you breathe. Exercise-induced asthma would not appear to fit into that category, but most atypical EIA reactions can be explained in physiological terms. The fact still remains that asthma symptoms will not be caused by anything unless the disease is already present. And we do not yet know what causes the disease.

There is no way of telling ahead of time what you will become sensitive to, and even determining your present asthma triggers can be difficult. Any given environment contains a number of things: you may enter a room containing cigarette smoke, a cat, and several women wearing perfume, and you may be handed an alcoholic drink and assorted canapés. If after fifteen minutes of this you begin to have trouble breathing and step outside for a breath of air, you may encounter pollen from trees, shrubs, and flower beds; molds; chemicals from distant factories; paint odors from newly decorated house trim, or gasoline exhaust from nearby traffic. Fortunately, chances are you will not react to more than a few of these triggers, and if you have had asthma for any length of time, you have probably identified the ones that are most serious for you.

Triggers, especially food allergens, are not necessarily constant; it is possible to eat a food without incident one day and to have a reaction on eating it a few days later. There are also a number of factors that may determine how severe your reaction is on any given occasion; alcohol, for example, lowers your allergic threshold and can increase the severity of an allergic reaction.

Since triggers develop only after exposure, you won't be sensitive to ragweed on your first encounter, but if you move into an area where ragweed grows, you may eventually, through repeated exposure, add it to your list of triggers. If you have never had a pet and someone gives you a dog, you may find yourself developing a dog allergy. It is this factor of developed sensitivity to new substances that makes the effort to find a more salubrious environment by moving to a different location so liable to fail.

Relocating to Get Away from Allergic Triggers

If you suffer from local, seasonal allergens, such as ragweed, or have a particular sensitivity, such as to dust mites, you may be tempted to relocate to a place that doesn't have them. Unfortunately, relocating rarely works.

Permanent Moves

Many people who regularly vacation in other areas and feel better there than they do at home think that that location would be beneficial. However, spending a short period in an area will not give a good reading on year-round conditions.

First of all, year-round climate conditions may vary widely. Dr. Craig Conoscenti, a respiratory specialist in Norwalk, Connecticut, tells of an asthmatic who moved from New Canaan to Tucson, where the mild winters had proved beneficial during vacations spent there. After all the expense and trouble of relocating, he found he had not reckoned with Tucson summers, which are very hot and made him extremely uncomfortable. Unwilling to experiment further, he moved back to New Canaan.

If the proposed new site is carefully researched to determine that the known allergens do not exist there—if you find an area where ragweed does not grow or dust mites do not exist, for example—it is possible that the initial reaction to the move would be greatly improved allergic asthma. Unfortunately, however, the nature of allergy is such that new allergies are liable to develop, either to new pollens and substances to which you have never been exposed before (for example, a New Englander encountering pine pollen in central California) or even to familiar substances that didn't use to bother you.

It is easier to understand why you acquire these new allergies if you realize that moving treats only the symptoms, triggered by substances to which you have been exposed for some time, and not the cause of allergic asthma (an overactive immune system).

An allergic European coming to America brings as part of his baggage his own group of allergens. Encountering ragweed (for the first time, since it does not grow in Europe) would create no problems for him, and he might think this was a great place to live free of allergy. However, if he were to relocate here, he might be disillusioned after a few years.

Vacations

If you have found that your allergies are particularly bad during a certain time of the year and you have a vacation spot where your asthma has customarily abated during your visits there, perhaps the best solution is not to relocate but to time your vacations for that period. Of course, if you have been going to your vacation spot in the winter and this change means going in September, you may encounter entirely different, and less favorable, conditions. But that would merely mean experimenting until you found a vacation spot that would work for you at the time you need to be away from your home area. This requires much less

─────── **Tips for Planning a Successful Vacation** ───────

As we have seen, having asthma should not interfere with your leading a normal life, including taking vacations. Planning is an important part of any successful vacation, and taking your asthma into consideration is no more difficult than planning what to pack. Anticipate possible problems and be prepared to deal with them.

1. *Take along extra medication and prescriptions.* Your doctor may suggest certain precautions or additional medication, depending on where you are going. Be sure you have enough of all medication with you, packed in different places. It is especially important to have a good supply on your person or in your carry-on bag if you are flying. Luggage can get lost, pocketbooks can be stolen, coats and jackets can be left behind. Also have prescriptions with you, and, if you are traveling out of the country, write down the names under which your prescriptions are available in that country. For example, cromolyn sodium is sold as Intal in the United States and Lomudal in Europe. If your doctor does not have this kind of information, call the Centers for Disease Control in Atlanta, Georgia, or ask if your local hospital has a travel clinic.

(A travel clinic, such as the one at Danbury Hospital in Connecticut, is a gold mine of information on such subjects as the injections advised for various parts of the world and even where to get local drugs when traveling. For example, a different malaria drug was recommended for each of three African countries to which an acquaintance of mine was going recently. The drugs were not available in the United States, but the clinic was able to suggest that they might be obtained at the London airport, during a short scheduled stop, and also to advise, if it was necessary to wait and get them on arrival in each country, what to take temporarily until that time.)

Inhalers and medications familiar to you are available worldwide, and many countries seem to be way ahead of the United States in this regard. As we have discussed, much of what Americans use was originally developed and used in Europe long before it was available here (and there are many effective drugs sold there that we still do not have access to). Sodium cromolyn, for instance, has been widely used abroad for many years and is possibly the most highly valued medication in England, though it still has not achieved wide acceptance here and usually takes second place to theophylline. Countries like India, too, which lack many of the amenities we are accustomed to, seem to be well equipped to deal with asthma even in some rather out-of-the-way places.

2. *Don't hesitate to go to a doctor abroad.* The American Embassy or any consulate will suggest one, and so will American Express, if you happen to carry that credit card. An American military base can also be helpful, and going direct to local hospitals can often be very satisfactory. Hotels usually have a list of local physicians who speak your language, and if you are on a regular cruise, there will be a ship's doctor on board. (If your picture of a ship's doctor is taken from stories by Somerset Maugham, you may be pleasantly surprised to encounter your own high-priced internist doing the honors, enjoying a working vacation, complete with his wife.)

3. *Investigate bed-and-breakfast accommodations carefully.* B&Bs are becoming increasingly popular, both here and abroad. They are generally much less expensive than hotels and motels, but accommodations vary considerably and need to be looked into in the usual way. In addition, anyone with asthma should ask about pets; the kind of congenial people who enjoy entertaining strangers in their homes are also often fond of pets. Exposure to cats and dogs, especially in the close conditions of a private home, is not a good idea and may rule out many potentially good B&Bs.

You might also ask about smoking. Ideally, a nonsmoking home would be most desirable but might be hard to find. Ask for a room as far as possible from the public rooms (dining and living rooms) to minimize secondary smoke.

Wood-burning fireplaces and stoves are sometimes a feature of country B&Bs. Pleasant as they are, they do emit a certain amount of ash and particles that may bother you. If you have found this to be the case, do not use the rooms containing them when the fire is burning. If you have already asked for a room away from the public rooms, you may not be bothered by smoke in your bedroom.

adjustment than a complete move and has the additional advantage of allowing you flexibility; a new allergy eventually acquired in the vacation site can be easily accommodated by a change of vacation locale.

Cruises   A generally successful vacation is a cruise, since being on the water reduces exposure to pollens, and the moist surroundings and less polluted sea air often make breathing easier. Even frequent stops in various ports don't last long enough for you to develop new allergies. Another advantage of a cruise is that even those who are considerably handicapped by their asthma can enjoy a wide range of activities in congenial company, rather than being confined to their home.

Of particular interest are cruises that include, along with the other passengers, special groups of people with asthma. The groups are under the supervision of respiratory specialists—doctors and nurses—and have access to oxygen, medicated treatments, and everything an asthmatic might require. It is a wonderfully secure and carefree way to experience all the fun of a cruise without worrying that you may have an attack or stand out by reason of your condition. You will be able to engage in any activity that appeals to you with no danger of unpleasant consequences if you happen to overdo it. And perhaps best of all, except for the members of your group, your shipboard companions will be regular cruise passengers, and the atmosphere will truly be a holiday one. (See Appendix 4 for further information.)

Types of Triggers

Allergens

What constitutes an allergen depends on individual reactions. The list of triggers on page 118 includes some common allergens (as well as other common triggers), and it appears that it is possible to become allergic to almost anything, including oneself.

It is estimated that at least one in every six people have allergies, including ten million asthmatics. And although there have been great strides in the treatment of allergic reactions, we still can treat only the symptoms, not whatever causes the body to generate them.

Food Allergies

As an increasing proportion of our food becomes processed and further and further removed from its natural state, we are exposed to additives, waxes, preservatives, and other nonfood ingredients that were unknown, or at least not so widely used, until fairly recently. We do not know what the effect of many of them may be after we have ingested them over a long period of time, but we do know, often from personal experience, that some, such as sulfites, can quickly make us ill, and after such an experience we try to avoid eating anything containing those ingredients. (See also Chapter 15, "Food and Asthma.")

Avoiding the food you are allergic to is not easy, however. If eating a strawberry gives you hives, or swallowing something made with eggs makes you throw up, the connection would seem to be obvious. But processed food isn't that simple. "Strawberry-flavored" foods may contain only synthetic flavors, not real fruit; eggs are often used for their binding and other qualities and may turn up where you have no reason to expect to find them. Reading the label is some help, and the FDA revises the labeling laws from time to time, giving consumers an opportunity to say what additional information they want to see.

Generally speaking, it is safest to eat as few processed foods as possible and to buy food products with the fewest ingredients listed on the label (not including the vitamins, which you should learn to recognize).

People often complain that they are allergic to their favorite foods—which is only to be expected, since you can be allergic only to something you have been exposed to, and once you develop a specific allergy, you are likely to become increasingly reactive to it. Doing without these foods is a hardship, but it is

Some Common Asthma Triggers

Air pollution	Nonsteroidal anti-inflamma-
Animals	tory drugs (NSAIDs)—"aspi-
Aspirin	rin substitutes"
Beef	Perfume
Beer and wine	Pollen
Down and other feathers	Shellfish
Eggs	Stress
Exercise	Sulfites
House dust	Viral infections
Milk and possibly other dairy	Weather
foods	Wheat
Molds	Yeast
MSG (monosodium glutamate)	Yellow food dye #5 (tartrazine)

better than getting asthma from eating them, and usually you can find other treats as replacements.

Airborne Allergens

Pollen is the most common allergen of this type and the one most people suffer from. It helps to know what pollens you are sensitive to, since they tend to be seasonal. Generally speaking, early spring brings tree pollens; early summer, grasses; and the fall, when "hay fever" sufferers usually have the most trouble, ragweed. Unfortunately, it is common to start out being allergic to ragweed pollen and end up, a few years later, allergic to trees and grasses, too. Pollen allergy is so common that many states issue daily pollen counts which can be heard on the radio during the season.

If you have this type of allergy, you may also react to flowering houseplants and bouquets of flowers.

Insect Bites and Stings

All summer long the newspapers contain stories of people who have died after being stung by a bee. A few years ago a neighbor was stung while gardening, and his wife came over to ask our help. He was in bed, turning all colors—blue around the lips, yellow under the arms and other lymph gland sites—and beginning to have trouble breathing. We gave him some antihistamine tablets and immediately drove him to the emergency room, where an Adrenalin injection counteracted the allergic reaction. In a few hours he was home, shaken by his experience but basically all right. And he had a new item in his medicine chest in case of future stings.

This can happen to anyone, even if you have been stung often without any ill effect. In fact, the more often you are stung, the more liable you are to eventually have a life-threatening reaction, although this is not invariably true. It is estimated that more people die of insect bites and sting reactions than from poisonous snake bites.

The danger of a fatal reaction to insect bites and stings has been known for thousands of years. Egyptologists, on translating the hieroglyphics on the tomb of a king who died in 2641 B.C., found that the cause of his death was a hornet's sting.

If you ever have any sort of extreme reaction to a bite or sting, such as considerable swelling and redness, check it out with a doctor. He or she may feel you should be prepared with a home kit in case you become more sensitive and have a serious episode.

Sometimes, of course, you can be bitten or stung by a poisonous creature, such as the black widow spider we have here in Connecticut or the scorpions of Florida. So between possible allergic reactions and possible poison, a bite or sting should always be monitored for a few hours. If you can describe the creature that bit you, correct diagnosis and treatment can quickly follow.

Airborne Chemicals, Insecticides, and Pesticides

These irritants can affect anyone, but because they are inhaled, they are even more serious for asthmatics. In our modern civilization they are ubiquitous, found in our homes, our gardens, and our environment. People with asthma should avoid aerosols, perfumes, spot removers (unless the chalk type), and many other household products. At least pay attention when something is used and see whether it bothers you.

Tobacco Smoke

Tobacco smoke is a potent pollutant that injures both the smoker and the nonsmoker. If you have asthma and smoke, you are not only adding to air pollution but you are sure to exacerbate your asthma. Most asthmatics know that tobacco smoke acts as a trigger, whether they themselves are smoking or they smell the smoke on the hair or clothing of someone who smokes or has been in a smoky environment, such as a meeting, seminar, or restaurant. More and more doctors are refusing to treat asthma patients who smoke unless they agree to give up the habit; they find it too frustrating to try to help those who will not help themselves.

Tobacco smoke is a complex mix of a number of harmful substances, including carbon monoxide, nicotine, and the insecticides and pesticides sprayed on the growing leaf. Not only are these substances irritating to the lung tissues but some of them cause undesirable physiological changes.

One of these changes of particular interest to someone who already has trouble breathing is damage to the delicate cilia in the airways. They lose their ability to clear out mucus, which instead clogs the passages where it becomes trapped and creates inflammation and even infection. A heavy smoker has fair warning that damage is being done when he or she hacks out the nonproductive "smoker's cough" on lighting up. Any cough is liable to precipitate an attack, but the tightness and wheezing of the chronic smoker's already oversensitized and constricted airways makes them especially hair-trigger.

Even in nonasthmatics smoking raises the blood pressure and increases the rate at which the heart beats. It also interferes with the lungs' ability to maintain the body's ratio between carbon monoxide and oxygen. The serum level of carbon monoxide increases and oxygen decreases, which, if the imbalance continues, can be fatal. At the very least, the effect on the heart is stressful and can lead to a heart attack.

Another unpleasant condition often caused by smoking is an increase in esophageal reflux or heartburn, which, in addition to interfering with sleep and with the enjoyment of food, can cause an asthma attack.

Another physiological, and possibly lethal, effect of smoking, as we have noted, is that it speeds up the metabolism of theophylline, which is often a maintenance drug, and of caffeine, to which theophylline is related. The increase in rate of metabolism resulting from the combination of a cup of coffee (more caffeine) and a cigarette, plus a maintenance theophylline tablet, can cause a sudden drop in the serum theophylline level, creating worsened asthma. If more theophylline is then given to counteract the attack, it may overcompensate, and potentially dangerous side effects may occur.

In addition to the damage smokers do to themselves, there are other people to consider. Secondary smoke—the smoke from other people's cigarettes that even nonsmokers inhale where tobacco is being used—is especially harmful to children. It has been proved that the effects of secondary smoke are similar to those of direct smoke, just as if the child or nonsmoking adult had done the smoking. And some studies indicate that the effects of secondary smoke may be even worse than those of direct smoke.

The effect of smoking on a fetus has been well documented; miscarriages and stillbirths are more common among maternal smokers, and so are low-birthweight babies. These statistics are especially daunting considering that the decrease in smoking among the general population in the United States does not extend to young women—the only group where smoking is on the increase.

There is no doubt that anyone with any degree of lung disease—or even with a family history of allergy or respiratory problems—should not smoke. In fact, an asthmatic should do even more than a healthy person to avoid secondary smoke. If you have stopped smoking and someone in your household smokes, you are still at risk. A cardiologist of my acquaintance had succeeded in quitting smoking, but his wife simply could not. He was convinced of the importance to his health of a smoke-free atmosphere, so he and his wife made a pact that she would smoke only in one room of the house, her den. Given the layout of their house, this has worked fairly well, and because of the restriction, she is smoking much less and may well give it up entirely one of these days. If you or someone in your household smokes and is having trouble stopping, ask your doctor for help. There are many tips and tricks that have been developed, and tobacco is so addictive that no one need be ashamed of needing help in learning to do without it. (See also pages 105–7.)

Minimizing Exposure to Triggers

Take triggers seriously. If you are sensitive to cats, spending just a few minutes in a room where a cat is allowed—even if the cat is not around at the moment—can cause an asthmatic reaction. Such short exposure may not have bothered you in the past, but your sensitivity can vary from one time to the next and you may at some point be in a particularly vulnerable state. It's better not to take the chance.

You cannot always know when you will be exposed to a trigger, but in many cases, especially in your own home and in familiar environments, you have some control. Aside from drugs that are used to prevent or control asthmatic reactions, regardless of what has caused them, there are certain steps you can take to minimize exposure.

Foods—the Elimination Diet

If a certain food you are allergic to is important to you, either in terms of nutrition or simply for pleasure, it may be possible to develop tolerance to it through a technique called the elimination diet.

One form of the elimination diet, in simplest terms, consists of cleansing your system of that particular food by not eating it for a period of time and then eating a very small amount of it. If all goes well, the amount is very gradually increased, and theoretically, the day comes when you can eat a normal portion without triggering an asthmatic attack.

A much more stringent variation of this procedure is also used by some allergists to determine what foods you are allergic to.

Do not attempt to use these techniques on your own; they must be set up and monitored by an allergist and require patience and discipline; there is no guarantee of success, since not all food allergies respond to this system.

Colds, Flu, and Other Respiratory Diseases

Anyone with a respiratory disease should try especially hard to avoid getting a cold. Since colds tend to be somewhat seasonal and to run through an area, most people are aware when "everyone has a cold." That is a good time to stay home and watch television instead of going out to a movie, and to avoid dinner parties or any large groups of people as much as possible.

If you have children, both they and you will unavoidably be exposed to whatever is going around. There is nothing you can do about it except practice the best possible hygiene—covering your nose and mouth when someone near you is sneezing, and washing your hands more frequently. Needless to say, keeping yourself fit, getting sufficient rest, and increasing your fluid intake will make you less susceptible.

If you do get a cold, don't treat it lightly. Take whatever steps are necessary according to how you feel and lie a little low until you have fully recovered. Do not hesitate to check with your doctor.

The flu is a more serious matter, and asthmatics are considered in the high-risk group, along with children, the elderly, anyone with a respiratory problem, and the people, such as teachers and nurses, who work with these groups. Most doctors recommend flu shots; check with your doctor before the flu season starts.

There is, however, one person who should never, under any circumstances, take a flu shot—that is anyone allergic to eggs. Flu vaccine is grown on eggs and and could cause a serious, even fatal, reaction if given to someone with an egg allergy. Since shots may be offered free at schools, district nurse offices, or community health centers as well as routinely at doctors' offices, it is essential that the allergic individual be aware of his or her own allergy and not count on others to think of it.

Flu shots are needed annually, and since there are many types of flu, the pharmaceutical companies try to anticipate what type will be prevalent in the coming season so that they can make that specific vaccine. Occasionally they guess wrong and the type of flu that goes around is not the type the injection protects against. Since flu shots are effective only before exposure, the high-risk group has no choice but to go ahead and get whatever is available before the season starts; fortunately, most of the time the vaccine will be effective.

Pneumonia

Another vaccine that is usually recommended for the high-risk groups mentioned above is the pneumococcal vaccine, which protects against one particularly virulent type of pneumonia. It is so well thought of that Medicare, which does not usually cover preventive medicine, makes an exception and covers this injection.

Only one such injection in a lifetime is usually recommended, so be sure you do not forget once you have had one.

House Dust

House dust might appear to be an avoidable trigger, but actually to avoid it entirely is almost impossible. There are, however, things you can do to minimize it.

It is currently believed that dust mites, which live in the dust, are the primary cause of dust sensitivity. In fact, the sensitivity is to the feces rather than to the mites themselves, but where there are mites there are feces, so the difference is not really of importance except from a scientific standpoint.

Dust mites are not found everywhere, and some parts of the United States—such as Denver—do not have them. They prefer a temperate but humid climate and do not tend to proliferate under extremely hot or cold conditions. Air-conditioning also seems to discourage them.

If you travel with a dust mite sensitivity, you may have more of a problem in some countries, such as Great Britain, and feel much better in others—for instance, Switzerland.

Of course, house dust is made up of many different things: bits of fabric, animal materials including saliva, feathers, pollen, and so on. Frequent dusting, preferably with a damp cloth, and vacuuming will help. It is best to be out of the house when this is done. If you must do it yourself, always wear a mask. The disposable white masks that come three to a packet can be found in most hardware stores; they can be used more than once providing you don't get them wet. If the elastic breaks, just staple it back on or replace it with a large rubber band.

Upholstered furniture, draperies, and rugs should be kept to a minimum. Wall-to-wall carpeting is especially undesirable; area rugs that can be sent out for periodic cleaning are less likely to be troublesome.

Pets

Among the most serious causes of allergic asthma are pets. One doctor I interviewed felt so strongly about it that he asked me to devote a whole chapter to explaining how important it is for asthmatics never to have any contact with cats. The difficulty is that people sometimes do not want to give up their pets even when told their dog or cat is contributing to their illness.

I witnessed this firsthand when my husband suddenly came down with severe asthma (he had had some episodes in childhood but very few as an adult) a month or so after I (in my pre-asthma days) brought home a stray kitten. Finally hospitalized with status asthmaticus, he admitted to his doctor that we had a pet cat. The doctor told him firmly that the cat would have to go, and in spite of his life-threatening attack, it was only with great reluctance that he finally agreed.

Fortunately, we were living in a sparsely furnished apartment, with no upholstered furniture, a few scatter rugs, and venetian blinds instead of draperies. The difficulty of getting rid of animal dander, skin scales, and other animal allergens is considerable, and studies have shown that even the most thorough cleaning, including washing walls and fabrics, is not enough for a very sensitive allergic person.

If you are allergic to pets, do not be surprised to find that sometimes a hotel room or lounge seems to bother you. Ask for another room and wipe your feet carefully before entering the new room. If you have had trouble in the past and are traveling by car, you might want to bring your own pillow and pillowcases.

While cats and then dogs seem to cause the most trouble, other pets, including guinea pigs and birds, can also be triggers. Larger animals, such as horses, are common allergens but easier to avoid if they bother you.

Sometimes otherwise intelligent people think that your allergic asthma is psychosomatic and that their pet will not make you sick if they put it in another room and don't tell you about it. When going to someone's house for the first time, ask about pets and keep this possibility in mind. Do not hesitate to ask again if you find you are beginning to have trouble breathing. It is better to leave a dinner party while you can still cope than spend the rest of the evening in a hospital emergency room because you didn't want to "make a fuss."

Other Animals

Most of the things we have been talking about so far are hazards we encounter indoors; many, like animals and airborne pollutants, may be present in both environments, and we may bring outdoor pollutants inside. If, for instance, we are very sensitive to animal dander, we may not associate an uncomfortable breathing episode that occurs when getting undressed at night with the fact that our shoes, socks, and clothing are full of dander from animals we met outdoors and petted or that rubbed against us. If we are not aware of this kind of problem, we can transfer the dander to the rug in our bedroom, the bedspread, or the sheets and pillows. At the very least, we may be depositing it on the easy chair we sink into to watch the evening news. It is exactly this sort of unwitting transfer of allergens and triggers that makes it so difficult to pin down what is bothering us. Our own awareness and observation are our best weapons and will be most helpful to the professional who is trying to analyze what is causing the asthma.

If you have found that you are especially sensitive to birds and animals, be careful when visiting zoos, farms, and similar animal habitats, and do not take up horseback riding. An aquarium might be a better choice for an outing than a place that brings you in contact with animals. Needless to say, domestic pets are not recommended for asthmatics; even if an allergy to them does not exist, it may develop from constant close contact.

Molds

The trouble with molds is not only that they are so ubiquitous but that there are so many hundreds of them; it is impossible to isolate the ones you are allergic to in order to become desensitized to those.

Mold spores are present in the air year-round and breed happily in any damp environment. Whether it is the grouting in your bathroom tiles, the foam mattresses and pillows you perspire on through a hot summer night, or the innards of your dehumidifier or air conditioner, you are liable to be subjected to mold formation throughout your house. Frequent laundering, cleaning, and airing are required, and chemicals, such as chlorine, that kill molds should be used, preferably in your absence. In addition, you will need to avoid secondhand book and clothing stores.

All air-filtering equipment, such as humidifiers and dehumidifiers, should be cleaned frequently with mold-destroying materials (Lysol, powders and liquids that contain chlorine). Washing with ordinary soap and water or even detergents won't remove or discourage mold.

It is important to remove mold as soon as possible after it has formed, not only so that your exposure is brief but also because it may eat into and destroy the material on which it forms and become impossible to remove.

If mold is a problem in your home or area, trial and error may help you arrive at the best materials. For instance, I always had trouble with shower curtains molding soon after I put up new ones. I tried cleaning them with Comet and a stiff brush, but it was harder each time and eventually there were black stains I couldn't completely remove. Shower curtains have gotten rather expensive, especially if you have to buy new ones every month, so eventually I tried just buying liners. To my surprise, I found the liners didn't mold as quickly—and I had bought inexpensive ones—so when they went on sale, I laid in a supply in the colors I needed and still have not had to replace my original ones. Even if they do eventually mold, you can buy six of them for the cost of one ordinary shower curtain.

Your best clue to the presence of molds, aside from the typical black and furry appearance, is their smell. If you once become aware of this, you can detect it and then distance yourself from unexpected encounters.

Air Pollution

It would not be healthful to feel confined to the house by air pollution; instead learn about this unfortunate fact of modern life so that you can reduce your exposure to it.

Insecticides   Obviously some places are more polluted than others, and you can quickly learn to recognize a restaurant or motel room or lobby that is hazy with tobacco smoke or has recently been sprayed with insecticide. Insecticide spraying in public places is usually done on a regular schedule, and if the restaurant, for example, is a neighborhood one, you might ask the proprietor what his spraying schedule is so you can eat elsewhere on that day and perhaps for a few days afterward.

Always notice whether you smell anything when you first enter a hotel or motel room. If it has been sprayed recently, the odor may be faint but the residue may be present on the pillows and bedding. You might not notice it until you go to bed and suddenly find breathing difficult.

An insecticide reaction can be serious (even for someone who doesn't have asthma but is sensitive to the chemical). A few hours spent with your head on the pillow of a room that has been sprayed that day might find you heading for the emergency room upon awakening. Do not hesitate to explain the problem to the manager. If the spraying is done on a floor-by-floor basis, all you may need is to be assigned a room on another floor. Most managers will be helpful (although once in a while you run into one who immediately thinks you are planning to sue him and will do whatever he can to persuade you to spend the night elsewhere, preferably after signing a disclaimer of liability on his part).

Other Air Pollution   Since air pollution can travel far from its source (as does smoke from forest fires and ash from an erupting volcano), you need to be aware that what you see around you is not a guarantee of what you are breathing. For instance, a big city, which usually has more polluted air than a less populated area, may spread its pollution to surrounding towns and villages, depending on which way the winds blow. Not only does the pollution retain its full strength but under certain conditions it may even increase.

It has been found, for instance, that air pollution originating in nearby New York City can create polluted air in Connecticut that is more harmful to the lungs than smoking two packs of cigarettes a day. Unfortunately, this is particularly true on just the beautiful, apparently clear, sunny days when you would be tempted to take a nice walk. The action of the sun on the polluted air, through the chemical reaction of photosynthesis, increases the pollution so that as the air travels from the city to Connecticut, it becomes even more harmful.

On days like this there is generally no sign of smog or even haze, but an asthmatic going for a brisk walk may experience considerable difficulty. Some states or areas issue daily air pollution bulletins, and the knowledgeable asthmatic listens for the "unhealthful" rating when there has been a particularly long spell of good weather. Occasionally a pollution alert, suggesting that anyone with respiratory problems stay indoors as much as possible, is issued over radio and TV stations.

Another kind of airborne pollution is smoke from factories, brush fires, power plants, and community incinerators. Now that it is recognized as unhealthful, burning leaves in the fall is banned by most communities, and though we may miss the haze we used to associate with autumn and the pleasant tang of this smoke, we are better for it. Industrial sources of smoke have proved more difficult to control in spite of existing laws; if you notice a smokestack spewing black smoke, do yourself and the environment a favor by reporting it.

Helpful Devices That May Minimize Triggers

Air Filters and Purifiers

House dust, pollens, and molds are airborne pollutants that can sometimes be effectively dealt with by air-cleaning devices, according to anecdotal reports from people who have used them (as reported to their doctors). Formal studies, such as the one referred to below, also tend to present a fairly positive view, even though it is equivocally stated because of lack of scientific proof.

It is estimated that in 1982 $150 million was spent on these devices, most of them small tabletop units retailing for $10 to $40. These small units tend to have limited capabilities, due partly to low air flow and the inability to effectively screen out allergens and pollutants with very small particles. If you find indoor air pollution a serious problem, you can try these inexpensive units for yourself, but if they are not satisfactory, you may want to investigate the two heavy-duty air filters described below. They are not inexpensive, and you should talk to your doctor and respiratory therapist before making a purchase; they may be able to tell you of experiences some of their other patients have had with one or the other, or they may recommend an entirely different device.

Inviracare   Molds are very difficult to deal with, and most air filter devices for the home are not effective against them. There is one, however, called Inviracare, that some respiratory specialists recommend. It comes in three sizes, with replaceable cartridges. There may not be a supplier in your immediate area, since only one is licensed in a state.

Hepanaire   This air filter device is also recommended by many pulmonary specialists. It uses the HEPA filter, described in an article in the October 1988 *Journal of Allergy and Clinical Immunology* by Dr. Harold S. Nelson and others as having been developed during World War II by the Atomic Energy Commission to remove radioactive dust from plant exhausts. This article, the report of a commission of specialists from around the country who studied types of domestic air-cleaning devices, stated: "The principal advantages of the HEPA filters are their unexcelled efficiency, which actually increases with use, and their lack of requirement for maintenance." In spite of these findings, the report, with true scientific caution, refused to make "any firm recommendations" for indoor air-cleaning devices because "the data presently available were inadequate to establish the utility of these devices in the prevention or treatment of allergic respiratory disease."

Air conditioners These are helpful against pollen because they filter the air coming in from outside and eliminate the need to open windows. The report referred to above noted: "It was regularly demonstrated that the rooms with either filtered or air-conditioned air contained lower pollen counts than rooms not fitted with these devices." Here again, however, it stopped short of a recommendation because "the extent to which this was true cannot be ascertained without the inclusion of a control group."

If your home does not lend itself to general air-conditioning, a window unit in the bedroom may provide a pollen-free night's sleep, and with a comfortable easy chair and a desk, the room can also be used for reading, working, and other daytime activities.

Negative-Ion Generators The demand for these has died out somewhat, since some of the devices "cleaned" the air but in the process left a large circle of black particles on the surface immediately around them and even on the walls. Other types clean the air by removing dust particles and may make you feel much better if you have one in your bedroom (a naturally dusty area) or any room where you spend a great deal of time. Unfortunately, they tend to deposit the dust on the walls, which should be vacuumed regularly, preferably in your absence.

Some electronic filters produce ozone, which is generally

irritating to asthmatics. Scan the literature and ask the dealer whether the device you are considering does this.

Charcoal-containing Filters These are most effective in removing tobacco smoke, but since you should not allow anyone to smoke in your house, and you can't very well carry one around with you, they are of limited use.

Other Filters With growing interest in breathing clean air and increased knowledge of the hazards of indoor pollution, new or improved devices are constantly coming on the market. Consult your doctor, respiratory therapist, or allergist as to what they recommend. Remember that what works for one person may not work for another, so trying out any new device of this sort is the only way you can find out whether it is for you.

Choosing Your Filter—Trial Periods There are many kinds of air filters and purifiers to choose from. If you are considering purchasing one of the expensive types, try to buy it with a short-term trial period so that it can be returned if it does not help your particular problem. If the dealer does not offer a trial period option, perhaps you can rent it for a month or two before committing yourself to buying it.

Masks

A number of years ago the inhabitants of Tokyo took to wearing masks when they went outdoors because the pollution was so severe. I do not know when this habit was discontinued, but it points up a simple preventive measure an asthmatic can take to cope with unexpected exposure to airborne pollutants and allergens.

Most hardware stores have a supply of masks, ranging from the simplest to the kind that are designed for spray-painting or exposure to seriously noxious fumes. The most popular appear to be the ones mentioned earlier, an inexpensive package of three lightweight white masks, attached to a rubber band that goes around your head. They are easy to pack for traveling and comfortable to wear, and I find them good protection at home when dusting, vacuuming, lawn mowing, and painting with water-based paints. You may not want to wear them in public, but a traveler who has them handy might just avoid a serious attack by doing so. One of the hazards of traveling abroad, for instance, is the fact that other countries allow smoking everywhere. European trains, planes, and public places will soon have you thinking that all Europeans are chain-smokers, and they aren't very sympathetic if you ask them to stop.

Ask your doctor or respiratory therapist for advice as to the best kind of mask, or masks, for you to have on hand. A lot depends on what you are sensitive to and how much the various triggers bother you.

Do not depend on a mask to make it possible to continue having a cat or other pet that causes a reaction; that kind of sensitivity is usually best controlled by getting rid of pets entirely. (A few people get themselves desensitized to a specific pet through injections. Ask your doctor whether he or she recommends this for you.)

Neck Gaiters

These soft, loose-fitting collars that look like the top part of a turtleneck can be used successfully instead of cold-weather masks. They are good-looking, come in many colors and fabrics, and don't attract attention. Worn comfortably around the neck, a gaiter will keep your neck warm and easily pulls up over your mouth and nose—and even ears—as soon as you go outdoors or if a wind suddenly comes up. If you have ever put a scarf or a handkerchief over your mouth on a cold day, you will find this much easier and more effective; it leaves your hands free and will not interfere with your breathing or get cold (as some masks do).

The first time you use a gaiter, you may be surprised to find you don't mind the cold at all and can take your usual walk without giving the winter weather a thought. Gaiters are used even by nonasthmatics when ice-skating or skiing.

Most ski and sports shops and some mail order catalogs, such as Lands' End, carry them.

13

Stress and Asthma

One of the most important recent advances in the treatment of asthma was the gradual realization by the medical community that asthma is not a psychosomatic disease. This conclusion was a long time coming for a number of reasons.

First of all, it is a chronic disease that is extremely variable; asthma triggers are numerous and vary from individual to individual. One person may have an acute attack on entering a room where a cat is sleeping; another may not be affected by a roomful of cats but will be sensitive to a moldy basement. And still another may cope with almost any indoor environment but start to wheeze when going out on a windy, wintry day.

Partly because of this variability and partly because of the nature of the disease, it has historically been difficult to treat. The frustration of many physicians trying to cope with asthmatics made it almost inevitable that some of them would throw up their hands and decide it was "all in the patient's mind."

It is only recently that medical science has been able to study the immune system and begin to understand the role it plays in asthma. Now the pendulum has swung all the way in the other direction, and asthma is now generally considered, as we have noted, to be caused by an overactive immune system. While this may be an oversimplication, it is a very encouraging development for asthmatics because it has led to more and more research aimed at treating the causes rather than the symptoms of this ancient disorder. Promising new medications aim to prevent as well as counteract bronchospasm and to decrease the incidence of acute attacks. At present, however, we are still grateful for steroids, bronchodilators, and all the other medications that make it possible to control acute episodes, prevent discomfort, and in most cases make it possible for asthmatics to lead normal lives.

The Role of Stress in Asthma

As we have learned more about the physiology of asthma, we have gained a greater understanding of the part played by the interaction between the mind and the body, and its effect on the immune system. Given the physical changes, such as constriction of the throat, that occur as a reaction to stress, it is obvious that being tense and anxious can also exacerbate the tightening of an asthmatic's twitchy airway muscles, thus creating a vicious circle; increased muscle spasm leads to greater difficulty breathing, which in turn creates greater anxiety, and action and reaction can easily turn mild discomfort into an acute episode.

If you do not have asthma, stress will not give you asthma, and no matter how stressed out you are, you will not have an asthma attack. If you already have asthma, stress can make it worse, and fear and anxiety may turn a little breathlessness into an all-out attack.

Coping with Stress

Every living thing is subject to stress; it is part of being alive. A plant may be stressed if you forget to water it. A mouse may be stressed if there is a cat in the house. Human beings live in a much more complicated environment and are bombarded with stimuli, situations, and schedules that are far more numerous and de-manding than they were in simpler times. Many of these stresses occur daily and are unavoidable.

Noise, for example, is stressful and frequently at such a high decibel level that deafness is increasing incrementally, especially among the young, and among workers in factories, airports, and construction. Earning a living is stressful; so are interpersonal relationships, having too much to do, or sometimes the opposite, being retired. Raising children and taking care of elderly parents are stressful. Sometimes just getting through the day is so exhaust-ing that we wonder how we are to continue managing. But while we cannot always control outside events, we can learn to modify our reactions to them. In other words, where we cannot avoid or lessen the things that cause stress, we can perhaps reduce the degree of stress they cause.

A person with asthma is subject to two kinds of stress that stem specifically from the disease, physical and psychological. The physical stress is created by bronchoconstriction, wheezing, mucus formation, and all the other familiar symptoms. Fortu-nately, today we can manage many, in fact most, of these with medications and treatment.

Psychological stress is more difficult, but it, too, can be managed, and since it is caused not only by asthma but also by the ordinary frustrations of modern civilization, learning to cope with it will improve our overall health and the quality of our life as well. Stress-reducing techniques help regardless of what is caus-ing the stress because they work from within.

Stress caused by asthma often takes the form of anxiety. If you have ever had a very bad attack, you will tend to be fearful of having another. You may not even be aware of this, but at the first sign of breathing difficulty or wheezing you may find yourself remembering what happened before and worry that it is going to happen again. Fortunately, if you have taken control of your asthma, you are prepared and know what to do—what medica-tions to take in what order, how to sit quietly, leaning forward slightly from the waist, in a position that gives your lungs maxi-mum room, how to slow down the tendency to breathe too fast by doing pursed-lip breathing (see Chapter 17), and whatever else your doctor and therapist have worked out for you. If none of the backup measures work, you are also confident that you can always get help, even if it means calling for an ambulance or going to the hospital emergency room. A great deal of freedom and support comes with the realization that it is all right to call on the experts when the situation is getting out of your control. Once you understand the nature of asthma and the progress of an attack, you know that trying to tough out an attack that is not responding to treatment is not being "in charge."

On the other hand, if you have gotten out of breath running for a bus, exercising without a warm-up period, going out on a cold, windy day, or eating too large a meal, you know that chances are if you keep calm and, if necessary, use your bronchodilator, you will be fine. Everyone gets out of breath under certain circumstances; you may do so a little more quickly than a nonasthmatic, but remember that not all breathlessness is asthma, and try not to get rattled. If you get anxious or panicky, your body will tense from those emotions alone and actually contribute physically to a worsening of symptoms. Of course, if your stress reduction techniques are not sufficiently developed and this should happen, the same rule applies as with any out-of-control asthma: Call for help.

Stress can be caused by another natural reaction—trying to hide the fact that you are having trouble breathing. Hiding it may mean not taking measures you normally would (doing pursed-lip breathing, using your inhaler, not talking), and not taking these steps plus worrying that you will get worse may prolong the episode. Start to notice how other people deal with problems that occur in public. We have all had frequent occasion to witness on television how celebrities and important public figures deal with an embarrassing situation. They usually pass it off with a smile or a wave and get on with their business.

It is best and causes least notice to handle this kind of situation in a matter-of-fact manner. Sometimes all you need to do is slow down. In a meeting, for instance, you might sit back and take a less active part for a while or excuse yourself and go and get a

Taking Your Asthma Public

Learn not to be self-conscious about having asthma. You may feel awkward when you need to use an inhaler or take medication when you are out in public or in a business situation, but you need not. If you proceed in a matter-of-fact manner to do whatever is necessary to take control of your asthma and do not act embarrassed or unduly alarmed, most people will take it for granted and hardly notice. Using an inhaler need not be a big deal, and if you are then able to calmly resume your conversation, meeting, or enjoyment of the concert, it will be no more remembered than if you had needed to use a handkerchief.

It is especially important for children to learn this and also to learn how to deal with the occasional teasing from other children. If a child can learn not to react to teasing and to matter-of-factly take two puffs and then get on with what he or she was doing, the teasing will cease to be fun and will tend to diminish and disappear. Sometimes it is even possible to turn the fact that the asthmatic child has special equipment into a plus, making the child important. Some children can carry this off very well, and others will always be shy and will need to be shown ways to minimize public exposure rather than capitalize on it.

Since many performers, speakers, and other people in public life who have obvious disabilities carry on as well as or better than the able-bodied, there are plenty of role models to encourage asthmatics to proceed with confidence. And the prevalence of asthma among top athletes who talk openly about their health problems is proof that this is not a disease anyone at any age must give in to or be embarrassed by.

drink of water. You can be sure you are not the only one in the room who has to take time out now and then; the more you take it for granted, the less attention anyone will pay.

I learned that lesson years ago from a client who was a very dignified and formal English gentleman. One day at a luncheon meeting he declined so many dishes that we all noticed, and someone finally asked if he was feeling all right. He calmly explained that his doctor had put him on an inconvenient but strict diet because he had been having a serious problem with flatulence. The conversation dealt briefly and a bit jocularly with the subject, and then we got back to talking business. The result was that no one paid any attention to the few times he had a problem, and neither he nor we were embarrassed as we all might otherwise have been.

So just relax and remember we are all human, and no one will think anything of your having a problem as long as you are coping with it and seem unconcerned.

Many specific techniques for dealing with stress have been developed through the ages. Some of them are described in detail in Chapter 14.

14

Stress Reduction Techniques

It is paradoxical that asthma, often in the past considered a psychosomatic disease and even today recognized as liable to be exacerbated by stress, frequently is treated solely by medication. For someone struggling to breathe, the immediate relief medication can bring is paramount, but it is now being recognized that stress reduction techniques, practiced regularly, may help reduce the amount and frequency of medication needed.

When control over your symptoms can be attributed partly to your own management of stress, you become more confident and relaxed, and a beneficial circle results. Stress reduction leads to more control, which leads to increased confidence and relaxation; this leads to less stress, which leads to less frequent symptoms, resulting in greater control, and brings you full circle.

Improvement that is primarily medication-related will not provide the same feeling of personal control and the sense that you have achieved greater health through your own efforts. Although asthma symptoms can be reversed through medication alone, underlying feelings of anxiety and fear of future attacks may not diminish, and any feeling of confidence may depend on access to your inhaler.

It is unfortunate that often no guidance is given by physicians as to how to utilize these stress reduction techniques, or what is known regarding their potential for mitigating asthma. There is even a tendency for some physicians to dismiss the benefits of treatment that is not medication-based, partly because it is not in their medical school core curriculum, and therefore they are not knowledgeable in this area, and partly because the results are less spectacular, less immediate, and less measurable than those achieved with medication. They are disturbed too by the possibility that these techniques may be substituted, inappropriately, for medication.

On the other hand, an increasing number of doctors not only are recommending these techniques but have even taken on the task of teaching some of them to their patients. Progressive relaxation and hypnosis, including self-hypnosis, both of which can be easily learned and taught by the physician, seem to be the most popular. If your doctor does not teach these techniques, perhaps he can recommend a professional who does. If not, your pulmonary rehab nurse/therapist or local hospital may have a list.

Stress and the Immune System

Much has been written about the negative effects of stress on overall health and on the quality of life, productivity, happiness, and even sex. But the most interesting relationship between stress and the human body, from the standpoint of the asthmatic, is its effect on the immune system. Dr. Ronald Glaser, Ph.D., an immunologist at the Ohio State University College of Medicine, has conducted studies that have shown that stressful events apparently reduced the immune system's ability to fight infection.

The UCLA medical school is in the forefront of research into the interaction of the brain, the endocrine system, and the immune system, under its program in psychoneuroimmunology and its positive as well as negative effect on illness. Although we have been aware since the time of Hippocrates that emotions can have a positive or negative effect on health, it was basically a theory arrived at by observation. Over the centuries the development of science tended to lead to the denigration of medicine based on anything but scientifically demonstrated evidence; observation, an important tool in diagnosis, was dismissed as largely "anecdotal." Today a scientifically acceptable body of medical research has established that negative emotions can affect the immune system and possibly make it more vulnerable to illness. What has been missing is scientific proof that positive emotions can have the opposite effect—that we can heal and make ourselves well through interaction with our immune system. This is the agenda of the UCLA program.

With any chronic disease stress and negative emotions directly related to the disease (in addition to the hassles of everyday life) are inevitable, but since asthma is considered an immune system disease, research that increases our knowledge about the effect of stress on the immune system is bound to be especially helpful to asthmatics. Among the leading researchers in psychoneuroimmunology are Dr. Ronald Glaser and psychologist Janice Kiecolt-Glaser (Ohio State University College of Medicine), who have demonstrated, through two studies of the effects of relaxation training on two entirely different age groups under very different kinds of stress, that the resulting enhancement of positive emotions also resulted in enhancement of the immune system.

In order to benefit from this new medical knowledge and to take charge of and control your asthma, you need to learn and practice stress reduction as well as the use of your medications. Remember, if your medical doctor's knowledge in this area is slight, rely on him as a highly specialized and valuable resource in his area, and seek, possibly with his help, equally good sources for the supplemental knowledge you need.

In investigating stress reduction techniques, you will find there are many options to choose from; the techniques that work best for you may not be the same ones that work for a friend. Also, it may take a couple of tries to find what you like and feel comfortable with. That is not a problem, since switching from one to another is easy, and after giving one a fair try, you should feel free to change if it is not satisfactory. Most people choose more than one; for instance, meditation and exercise make a good combination.

Where to Start—Pulmonary Rehabilitation

Whatever else you decide to try, start with pulmonary rehabilitation. This is not really a stress reduction technique (it is much more than that), but joining a pulmonary rehab group certainly reduces stress, and it opens the door to everything you need to know and do. Pulmonary rehab nurses and therapists will teach you as much about your asthma as you want to know (some people prefer to skip the anatomy). They will patiently show you how to use your inhaler properly (this is not easy—many people never really listen to instructions or forget to follow them after a few days), explain the function of your various medications, and if your doctor hasn't already done so, introduce you to such devices as spacers and peak-flow meters.

A pulmonary rehabilitation program is usually part of a hospital pulmonary department. Do not depend on your doctor to suggest joining one, or even necessarily to be aware of its existence.

To find the program nearest you, look at the list in Appendix 5. If none is listed in your area, check with your state American Lung Association (Appendix 3); new ones are being established all the time.

What Is a Pulmonary Rehabilitation Program?

Although it may differ slightly from hospital to hospital, a pulmonary rehab program provides rehabilitation for, and improves the health of, those with pulmonary problems. It is administered by a team of health professionals and generally consists of a pulmonary nurse specialist, a respiratory therapist, and a medical pulmonary physician who serves as an adviser. Your own doctor is still in charge of your case, and the team supplements and expands his care, just as a physical therapist works hand in hand with an orthopedic surgeon.

Additional team members may include a psychiatric nurse clinician, a nutritionist, and physical and occupational therapists; often one team member will function in several areas.

What Does a Pulmonary Rehabilitation Program Do?

While no two programs are exactly alike, all have the same basic goal: to teach you how to manage the specific problems that having asthma creates. The program includes a personal support system and education about all the various aspects of asthma, including stress reduction techniques and exercise.

Throughout your association with the program you will always have someone to answer your questions, and your health and progress will be constantly monitored and evaluated. You will be taught not only what exercises to do but also how to do them. You will learn the importance of a peak-flow meter and how to use it and, if prescribed, a home nebulizer, portable oxygen, and similar equipment.

If you are considering buying a dehumidifier or a humidifier, you will be able to discuss the latest findings as to the pluses and minuses of doing so and can bring to your sessions all the other questions that you may not feel comfortable trying to discuss with your doctor.

What Has Pulmonary Rehab to Do with Stress Reduction?

You will experience stress reduction as soon as you join a pulmonary rehab program. The support of these health professionals and their confidence in your ability to improve yourself creates an atmosphere entirely different from that of a doctor's office.

As you can see, your active participation in your own health is the key; how much you benefit from what you learn is entirely up to you. And being surrounded by so much encouragement, caring, and support helps you help yourself.

Breathing Exercises for Stress Reduction

Breathing exercises, best learned in a pulmonary rehab program, are discussed at some length in Chapter 17. They are mentioned here because they are an important part of stress reduction for someone with asthma and are possibly the first kind of exercise you will be taught.

Other Relaxing Exercise and Activities

First of all, notice we say "exercise and *activities.*" Aerobics and jogging have been so visible in recent years that most people don't think they are benefiting unless what they are doing is fairly strenuous. But what we're interested in here is reducing stress, and that doesn't require strenuous aerobics at all. In fact, Dr. William P. Morgan at the University of Wisconsin includes relaxing in an easy chair among stress-reducing activities. To make it work, you also have to think happy thoughts or imagine being someplace that gives you pleasure.

A famous nineteenth-century writer once described his protagonist's way of relaxing: he would go to the zoo and look at the elephants. The size, slow movements, and apparent serenity of the huge creatures had a calming and relaxing effect on him. Many people find they can achieve a calm and relaxed state by going out on a clear moonless night and looking at the stars. And a study, again at the University of Wisconsin, found that for many people taking a shower reduced tension (this might work particularly well for someone with asthma, since a hot shower relaxes muscle spasm, and the warm moist air is often beneficial).

The study that documented the tension-reducing effect of taking a shower also included a test of four different walking speeds. Results showed that stress reduction occurred just as completely by walking slowly as by walking fast. And instead of the twenty-minute minimum needed for heart-healthy aerobic exercise, relaxation was achieved with a much shorter exercise time.

The relaxing effect of a stroll is enhanced considerably if you can take it in pleasant surroundings; a walk in the woods or along a beach is better than one on a busy city street. But as long as you enjoy the walk, it is an activity almost guaranteed to relax you regardless of where you do it.

Take the same easy approach to other activities that give you pleasure. Cycling can be relaxing, even if you do it on a stationary bike. It's very important to have a comfortable seat if you are going to enjoy this activity, and many modern bike seats are surprisingly uncomfortable. If you are planning a bike purchase, whether stationary, mountain, or other kind of bike, check out the seat by actually sitting on it and cycling for a few minutes.

If you want and are able to exercise for fitness, you will have to go to a more strenuous level. See Chapter 16 for heart-healthy, working-up-a-sweat exercises.

Meditation and Other Relaxation Techniques

Meditation

About twenty years ago meditation burst on the American scene through a group called transcendentalists who taught transcendental meditation. Practiced by monks in the Far East since ancient times, meditation soon had many adherents in this country because of its claims to improve health, including lowering blood pressure.

At first many experts questioned these claims, but eventually serious medical tests were conducted and found they were valid. There is still some question whether the physiological benefits of meditation, such as lowered blood pressure, last if meditation is discontinued, but no one denies it is beneficial and successful in reducing tension and anxiety.

In my own experience, I have found that meditation really works and is very calming. It gives you perspective and somehow establishes a distance between you and your problems and anxieties, so that they do not have the same emotional impact and you can view them more objectively.

You can learn to meditate from books (they are easily found in libraries) or from a teacher; if you have a choice, a teacher is better. For one thing, meditating with someone else reinforces your own experience. I am not inclined to the mystical, but there is no denying the enhanced effect of group meditation. Since you will probably do it alone most of the time, it is helpful to start with a teacher, and perhaps a group—probably you will learn more quickly under those circumstances.

One of the things books may not tell you is not to try to evaluate whether you have had a "good" meditation or whether it is working. Go with the procedure and do it without distraction for the fifteen or twenty minutes suggested, and then simply go about your life. Do it twice a day if possible, and give it a fair trial by sticking with it for a couple of weeks.

It is very pleasant and requires no equipment aside from a comfortable place to sit that will enable you to keep your back straight. You don't even need a very private place in which to meditate, since minor distractions, such as someone turning on the radio, are simply accepted into your environment without stress.

Progressive Relaxation, or Relaxing All Over

There are many variations on this technique, but all of them are based on separating out muscle groups and relaxing them one at a time, starting at your head, until you have consciously relaxed your whole body.

You do this by lying down or sitting in a chair with your eyes closed and concentrating, for instance, on your facial muscles and on relaxing them. The way to do this is to tense them first for several seconds and then relax them for half a minute. This sequence makes it possible to tell the difference between the two states and to realize when they are relaxed. Once you know what relaxed muscles feel like, you will be able to achieve that feeling by consciously relaxing them.

It is easier to learn if someone in your pulmonary rehab program talks you through it by softly telling you which muscles to relax and suggesting how good you are feeling as you proceed. There are also tapes you can buy to talk you through this exercise, and they are very soothing and pleasant to work with. Don't be surprised if you nap briefly when you are finished. You will wake up quite refreshed.

Hypnosis and Self-Hypnosis

Most of us have never encountered hypnosis in any serious context, but it has a long tradition. It was used medicinally by the early Persians and the gurus of India, and records have been found in writings of the ancient Egyptians and Greeks. Hypnosis became a fashionable fad in late-eighteenth-century France when a Viennese physician named Franz Mesmer (hence mesmerism) claimed he could cure disease by utilizing the "vital magnetic fluid" in the human body. Louis XVI—caught between the protests and complaints of the medical profession, who thought Mesmer was a charlatan, and his numerous patients and admirers (including Marie Antoinette, Madame du Barry, and the Marquis de Lafayette)—appointed a commission, headed by Benjamin Franklin, to look into Dr. Mesmer's claims of cures. The report of the commission was surprising; it did not ascribe the cures to Mesmer's theory of "animal magnetism," but it did agree that he had effected genuine cures in many instances. As to the explanation of these cures, the commission said it thought they were due to mass hysteria and the "imagination." Mesmer continued to be ridiculed by doctors and scientists of the time, and mesmerism fell temporarily out of favor.

Surprisingly enough, it surfaced again in nineteenth-century

England, where a surgeon named James Braid became interested in it, though without the magnetic fluid concept, and coined the term "hypnotism" to describe the process of creating a highly suggestible trance state in his patients. This time it became incorporated into standard medical practice and was studied and used by physicians throughout Europe.

Today hypnosis is an accepted if sometimes controversial procedure, and is studied and experimented with by serious scientists. It has been used successfully in the treatment of people with asthma, primarily as a relaxation technique, although some physicians believe it has beneficial physiological effects and even enables an asthmatic to control bronchial constriction, relaxing the spasm and, to some extent, opening the bronchial tubes. Since a patient under hypnosis is very suggestible (providing the suggestion is not contrary to his code of behavior), it has been possible to suggest that breathing will improve as one relaxes. Studies done in England by Dr. Margaret Turner Warwick at the University of London gave positive results when hypnotized patients were compared with a nonhypnotized control group.

Self-hypnosis operates on the same principle, except that the physician teaches the patient how to induce a kind of hypnotic state in himself. In the process the undesirable symptoms are visualized and discarded, and the visualization then turns to pleasant imaging that creates a relaxing atmosphere. Not everyone can do this successfully, but it is worth trying if you like the idea. Be sure the hypnotist is a pulmonary physician or a physician/hypnotist recommended by your doctor or pulmonary nurse/therapist. Generally, once you have been trained, you will do it twice daily, once in the morning and once in the evening, along with progressive relaxation, as part of a preventive regimen.

Although in itself hypnotism is not dangerous and the trance state is not at all fearsome, there is a risk that you may think you feel better when that is not physiologically the case. A physician/hypnotist or a pulmonary therapist who checks your condition directly after a session by using a peak-flow meter can soon determine whether your improved state is physical or euphoric, and proceed accordingly. There is certainly benefit in feeling better even if you still have to rely on medication. The purpose of hypnotism is not to replace medication but to gain greater control of and reduce asthma symptoms. The general consensus among physicians who look favorably on hypnotism seems to be that it is useful in stress reduction and in inducing relaxation, which in turn can help your asthma.

Not everyone is a good subject for hypnosis, although most people can be hypnotized, even if not deeply. Self-hypnosis is usually a pleasant and interesting skill, provided you are trained by a recognized medical expert working with your doctor. It is not something you should try to learn on your own from a book.

Biofeedback

This technique has been used successfully in helping patients to achieve a great deal of control over physiological conditions and to actually change them. It generally requires that you work in a laboratory with equipment that measures your skin temperature, degree of muscle relaxation, and similar physical conditions. The screen records the results of your efforts to change a specific physical function, and as you watch what is happening you develop a sense of how to achieve this goal even without a screen, and deliberately controlling specific physical reactions becomes possible. Usually the first thing you learn is how to raise your skin temperature and lower your blood pressure. It is very exciting to find yourself controlling these usually autonomous happenings, and the experience should counteract the feeling of helplessness that sometimes accompanies asthma as well as give you confidence in your ability to exert some measure of control over your disease.

The application of biofeedback to asthma usually targets the airway muscles; the goal is to teach the patient how to voluntarily relax them so that the airways can open up and allow breathing to become easier. This is apparently much more difficult than controlling skin temperature and has had limited success so far.

There is a recent theory that relaxing the facial muscles seems to reduce the contraction of the airway muscles, and that, conversely, the airway muscles tend to tense as the facial muscles tense. Another development is a device that helps the patient distinguish between tight and relaxed airway muscles by listening to the nature of the breathing sounds. Some scientists say this approach, which eliminates the need for costly equipment, not only has succeeded in helping asthmatics to feel better but also has led to a decreased need for medication.

Biofeedback is a completely safe, widely accepted, and noninvasive technique. It is generally most successful when combined with other relaxation techniques, but people differ in their ability to master it and you may not find it helpful. Ask your doctor to suggest a resource in your area where it is available.

A Positive Attitude

Some years ago Norman Cousins wrote a book called *Anatomy of an Illness* about how he had cured an "incurable" disease after doctors had given up on him. He had developed the theory that the mind could help marshal the healing resources of the body to combat and even cure illness. In his book he described in detail his experiences and his incredible recovery. If you want to know how he did it, read his book (it's easy reading). If you wonder how sound his theories are, I can only say that they are now so widely accepted that he received the only honorary degree in medicine ever awarded at the Yale University School of Medicine by the New Haven County Medical Association and the Connecticut State Medical Society. He is a board member of the Center for Health Communication of the Harvard School of Public Health and the Institute for the Advancement of Health. He is also presently adjunct professor at the UCLA School of Medicine.

Mr. Cousins's most recent book, *Head First: The Biology of Hope,* reflects his experiences over the past ten years in the medical community, where he has had the opportunity to explore the mind/body connection and the effect of a positive attitude on speeding recovery from illness, bolstering the immune system, and even, possibly, creating greater resistance to disease; although this has never been "proved," it has been confirmed by numerous scientific observations and studies.

As usual, however, the tendency to go overboard on new discoveries has led to extreme statements. Articles in popular magazines sometimes give the impression that people who get cancer, for instance, have only their poor mental attitude to blame. Someone who is sick does not need the added burden of feeling that it is all his or her fault, and such interpretation of the positive attitude approach is a distortion of what it actually means.

It does appear that a pessimistic attitude, stress, a lack of the will to live—whatever form of negative reaction a person brings to illness—do tend to exacerbate problems and possibly do affect the functioning of the immune system. As we have noted, doctors have always spoken of patients who "fight to stay alive" and who have a "strong will to live" as having a better chance to achieve their goals than patients who give up and feel hopeless. And almost everyone knows or has heard of elderly patients who have simply "willed" themselves to die.

Asthma, like all chronic diseases, can get rather tiresome when it is in an active stage, and it is unquestionably difficult to be cheerful when you are having trouble breathing. But since we know that relaxing has a specific and important role in reducing muscle spasm, and since a positive attitude makes it more likely that you will stick to your exercises and work to get yourself in the best possible physical condition (which will in turn automatically make you feel more cheerful and self-confident), it is obviously important to try to emphasize the positive as much as possible.

It is a known fact that it takes more muscles to frown than to smile, but it is only recently that physiologists have discovered that just putting a smiling expression on your face, even if you aren't really smiling from pleasure, causes your body to react chemically to create feelings of euphoria and cheerfulness.

Even just using negative words has a negative effect, and everyone tends to react positively to positive words. For instance, many advertising copywriters know that "but" tends to turn off readers, while "and" carries them along with you; most ads and commercials try to avoid a "but," even if introducing a negative about a competitive product. Peggy Noonan, Ronald Reagan's speechwriter, in an article in the *New York Times* magazine section, told how the president never objected to words and phrases in his speeches *except for eliminating any negative words.* For instance, she was told not to write "I would never say . . ." but instead to go with the positive "I always say . . ." Reagan was clearly aware of the value of, and tried to maintain, a cheerful, amiable, positive attitude, and if Norman Cousins is right, this may be one of the reasons why, although well along in years, he has experienced remarkably swift recoveries from operations and even from an attempted assassination.

We do know (in the scientific sense) that a negative attitude can make us ill. Why shouldn't it then be feasible that a positive attitude can give us a better chance of being well? And if it doesn't, we will certainly have made life much more enoyable for ourselves and those around us.

Applying Stress Reduction Techniques

Although people often resist taking medication, sometimes to the point of cutting back on it themselves without consulting the doctor, at present it is an essential part of successful asthma management. It cannot be emphasized too strongly that stress reduction techniques are not a substitute for medication; they are best used in conjunction with it. If you try to use them when you should be calling on medication, you may allow the episode to progress to a much more serious stage that will be harder to reverse.

On the other hand, none of these techniques are the least bit dangerous or unpleasant, and the result of learning to use them can be very rewarding. You should at least see what they can do for you. If by any chance they help reduce the amount of medication you need, you will do away with many of its undesirable side effects and, given the high cost of prescription drugs, may reduce your drugstore bill appreciably. In addition, stress reduction is a skill that will help you not only mitigate asthma but also cope with the many small hassles and problems of daily life. And best of all, you will have accomplished it yourself.

15

Food and Asthma

If you have asthma, there are two aspects to food that are of special concern: one is nutrition, the role of food in maintaining a healthy immune system and contributing to overall health; the other is your own personal food triggers, those foods that may cause asthma symptoms due to allergy or special sensitivities on your part. What constitutes a good diet, as far as we know today, is basically the same for most healthy people, but the foods that trigger asthma symptoms are not the same for everyone. Although certain foods are more liable to be troublesome, and some food additives have more of a history than others of causing asthma symptoms, you personally may be able to eat many of them without any ill effect. Just as there is no predicting what you may be allergic to, there is no telling what foods you should avoid, and even the fact that a parent or a sibling reacts to a specific food does not mean that you will.

Nutrition

It sometimes seems we are more concerned about what kind of fuel we put in our cars than about what we put in our bodies. Since human fuel, or food, greatly influences our health and well-being, why is this so? Perhaps we get discouraged because solid information is hard to come by; even nutritionists and scientists disagree, and consumers are confronted with conflicting claims and frequent "new" (and often contradictory) findings. The media, over-eager to disseminate information because of the need for "news," publicize even small, statistically nonsignificant studies as if they proved something, and food manufacturers fill supermarket shelves with confusing health claims (as when "No Cholesterol" is prominently displayed on a food product, such as vegetable oils, that could never possibly contain cholesterol, regardless of brand).

The best we can do is try to eat a well-rounded diet. Unfortunately, this is not easy.

A Well-Rounded Diet

There is no magic formula for achieving this worthy goal. The starting place is knowledge of what nutrients we need in what quantities, and what foods contain them. Unfortunately, this kind of knowledge is unattainable.

The question of what nutrients we need is in many important areas still unknown and in others very controversial. The RDAs (recommended dietary allowances) and the USRDAs (United States recommended daily allowances; see pages 162–63 if you are not sure what these are) are both too generalized to be a real guide, and they are lacking in many important nutrients. It is only recently that there has been any mention of trace elements, yet we do know that very small amounts of some nutrients are truly essential. Selenium, long thought to be commonly deficient in Americans, has just now been added to the USRDAs, and the USRDA for vitamin C has recently been increased, but only for a small, specific group. Many Americans routinely take amounts of vitamin C well over even this guideline and other antioxidants as well.

As to what foods contain what nutrients, the answer to that question is much more variable than the Department of Agriculture's Composition of Foods data base would have you believe. Take the potato, for instance. It is usually said to be a good source of vitamin C; what no one tells you is that that depends on when it was harvested (compared to when you eat it) and whether it is raw, cooked, or processed. Here is how it varies:

Mean Total Vitamin C Content in Potatoes Harvested in Autumn and Sampled Periodically

	Raw	Fresh, Peeled, Cooked, and Mashed	Reconstituted Flakes
October	29.3 mg.	18.8 mg.	8.0 mg.
February	11.7 mg.	8.2 mg.	3.1 mg.
May	10.6 mg.	6.8 mg.	2.1 mg.

(Source: U.S. Plant, Soil and Nutrition Growing Laboratory, Ithaca, New York.)

In other words, depending on when you eat it, a raw potato may contain from 29.3 mg. of vitamin C to only 11.7 mg. six months later. The same thing is true, to a greater or lesser extent, of oranges and all other fruits and vegetables.

The solution in this case is to do what our great-grandparents did—eat fresh foods in season. Or take advantage of the best of modern food processing and eat frozen foods out of season (but not potatoes if you are sensitive to sulfites, unless you read the label—see pages 166–69).

Another thing you can do is not take all of this too literally. Even with all the confusing information being fed the consumer, it is possible to have at least a rough idea of how to plan a balanced diet. And to make this task a little easier, be aware of the

RDAs; just think of them as an indication of what you need, and be grateful that they are updated approximately every five years to incorporate new nutritional discoveries.

The RDAs and the USRDAs The RDAs—developed by the National Academy of Sciences—are broken down into twenty-six groups, including age and sex, and are supposed to be the nutritional requirements of "healthy" people. Fortunately, having asthma doesn't mean you are necessarily unhealthy, just that you have to try a little harder to keep your immune system at its best and to avoid your food triggers and sensitivities.

The nutrient lists on food packages, however, are not RDAs; they are a compacted list (usually only seven nutrients are included) of USRDAs, which are derived from the RDAs. (Unfortunately, important information is left out in an effort to keep the list short enough to fit on the package.) People tend to take these lists very seriously, but many critics feel they are far too rough a guide to be useful.

Instead of the RDAs' twenty-six age groups, the USRDAs use four: pregnant or lactating women, infants of up to one year, children under four years, and adults and children over four years. You can see from these groups that the USRDAs make no distinction between the dietary requirements of a five-year-old boy and a ninety-five-year-old woman, though obviously their nutritional needs are quite different. And though the USRDAs are compiled from the highest values of the RDA tables, many nutritionists consider the requirements far from adequate. Many knowledgeable consumers now routinely use the listings as a sort of baseline and try to get more of certain nutrients, such as vitamins C, E, and B, and minerals, such as zinc and iron, depending on their age and sex and the latest news about nationwide nutritional deficiencies.

Another problem with the food package lists of percentages of USRDAs is that the lists do not distinguish between the nutrients found naturally in the foods and those added as supplements. Single foods do not naturally provide 100 percent of the USRDAs, so food manufacturers who advertise that their foods do make up the difference by adding vitamin supplements. Since supplements added to processed foods are not designed for each individual's need in terms of amount or kind, individual requirements may still be lacking in a given food. In addition, *The FDA Consumer,* a government publication that contains news of FDA rulings and articles on nutrition, indicates that the government does not recommend vitamin and mineral supplements (although it actually endorses them to some extent, as when it allows vitamin D–enriched milk and does not object to vitamin supplements and mineral supplements added to "enriched" foods). In spite of this, foods are advertised as providing total nutrition (as defined by the USRDAs), and you may find it difficult to tell, even if you read the package, which are the nutrients found in the food and which are due to added supplements.

If you find USRDA vitamin and mineral supplements added to food a convenient way to get baseline nutrition, there is no great objection to it, provided you understand its limitations. You could, however, do just as well less expensively by eating cereal or other food that has not been enriched to this extent and taking your customized vitamins separately, either in your food or through supplements. Adding your own vitamin supplements to your diet will also give you a much wider choice of foods.

The Dietary Goals

Another guideline the government offers suggests that you eat more complex carbohydrates, less refined and processed sugar, and less fat. The goal most people have trouble with is the limitation on fat consumption. Suggested fat intake, for example, is limited to 30 percent of daily calories—10 percent saturated fat, 10 percent monounsaturated fat, and 10 percent polyunsaturated fat. (The fat recommendation is often distorted when it is described as "no more than 10 percent saturated fat." The implication is that the recommendation is to eat more of the other two fats, but this is not the case.)

While it is true that saturated fat, rather than dietary cholesterol, has been implicated recently in contributing to plaque formation and therefore heart disease, the dietary goals still suggest that the healthful thing to do, as noted, is to reduce intake of all fats to 30 percent or less of your daily calories. Given the potential effects of a high polyunsaturated fat intake (including early signs of aging, shortened life span, increased early wrinkles, and similar undesirable possibilities), hedging one's bets might seem to be the healthiest course. Theoretically, if you feel the need for more fat, monounsaturated (olive oil or canola oil, for instance) is the safest one to increase.

Food Groups

A third guideline to healthier eating is the "Basic Four" food groups. These Basic Four are:

1. the milk group
2. the meat and fish group
3. the vegetable and fruit group
4. the bread and cereal group

You can eat a balanced diet, within the so-called dietary goals, if you choose one item daily from each group (you may substitute one item for another in the same group). With this guide you will theoretically get both variety and a good nutrition mix.

You can find this information, listing specific foods and allowable quantities in each group, in a number of inexpensive paperback books on nutrition. In addition, a particularly handy and attractive four-color poster, with detailed Basic Four information, is offered by the Center for Science in the Public Interest in Washington, D.C. It lists many foods you might never think would be allowed and provides for great variety. Once you become familiar with the groups and the allowable amounts, it won't be necessary to constantly consult a list; as long as you are in the ballpark, and provided your health is good, you may not need a rigid regimen.

What About Supplements?

The question often arises as to whether there are any vitamins or minerals thought to be especially helpful in reducing asthma. At present there do not seem to be any that are widely recommended, although a number of studies seem to suggest some progress in that direction. The *Annals of Allergy* reported a study in which children with asthma were apparently helped by B_6 supplements, and vitamin C has also had some favorable reports. In addition, studies described in the *Journal of the International Academy of Preventive Medicine* found that a combination of calcium, vitamin D, and vitamin A, given to approximately ten thousand patients, reportedly reduced the severity of the asthma of more than three quarters of the group.

These results would need to be replicated by additional studies to be considered definitive; so far none has led to recommendations of any specific supplement regimen for those with asthma, but research is ongoing.

An Asthmatic's Special Concerns

A person with asthma has to pay attention to dietary factors that need not concern other people. The three most important are allergens, sensitivities, and food/drug interactions. The first two may bother a person whether or not he or she has asthma but will not cause asthma in a person who does not have the disease; the latter is inherent in the drug, regardless of the person taking it.

Food Allergies

Food allergies and food sensitivities are usually considered separately although even doctors do not always agree on what category a food reaction falls into.

The most difficult thing about food allergies is not avoiding the troublesome foods (although this can be very difficult) but discovering which cause your allergic reaction. Food allergies are

liable to change or vary in degree of sensitivity from day to day
and from season to season. For instance, I can drink milk in the
winter (presumably because I am not reacting to pollen), but not
when my hay fever is active. If in the middle of the winter I am
exposed to an allergen, such as a very moldy environment, without realizing it, I temporarily cannot tolerate even a cup of yogurt,
which doesn't usually bother me even in ragweed season. Of
course, this may be due to a lactase deficiency (a food intolerance
rather than an allergy), but it is definitely worse if I am already in
an allergic state.

If the allergic reaction is strong, such as vomiting or hives or
itching, it will usually be fairly easy to isolate what caused it. Since
avoidance is the only real treatment, try to notice if your asthma
seems to get worse during or soon after eating (although in fact
the reaction may not take place immediately) and make a list of
what you ate. After a couple of such incidents you may be able
to figure out what you're allergic to. This may not work with
restaurant meals, where you are exposed to other potential triggers such as smoke, insecticides, perfume, and unknown ingredients used in food preparation.

Your pulmonary physician will probably not want to get very
deeply involved with the allergic triggers of your asthma and may
suggest you consult an allergist. Unfortunately, some allergy tests
for food are controversial and, unless the reaction is clear-cut, not
always conclusive.

Sensitivities

As noted, a distinction is made between allergies and sensitivities, but from your standpoint the reactions are much the
same, and so is the treatment. One of the most ubiquitous sensitivities is to sulfites.

Sulfites   Sulfites are used in foods and drugs as preservatives, to
prevent browning (as of cut vegetables and fruits), to inhibit bacterial formation, to control fermentation, and as antioxidants.
Their safety was first questioned in 1907, but it was not until 1986

that the FDA finally passed a limited ban, preventing their use on raw packaged or unpackaged fruits and vegetables. Ironically, one of the exceptions was potatoes, in spite of the fact that the ban was initiated partly as a result of the death of a ten-year-old girl with sulfite sensitivity who unwittingly ate sulfited french fries in a restaurant after having been assured that the potatoes had not been treated with sulfites. (The restaurant had no way of knowing—the package they came from had not been properly labeled.)

In the spring of 1990 the FDA announced a further ban on "the use of sulfites on fresh potatoes because of severe allergic reactions to these preservatives." There have now been four deaths attributed to eating sulfite-treated potatoes in restaurants. According to the FDA, ". . . up to a million asthmatics may be

---

Common Foods That Often Cause Allergic Reactions

These are foods that are good and wholesome in themselves but seem to be more allergenic than others. The list is by no means complete, but it may offer a clue to the cause of the problem if you have an allergic reaction after eating.

Beef If beef is an allergen, you may also be allergic to veal.

Chicken   If chicken is an allergen, you may also be allergic to eggs.

Chocolate   If chocolate is an allergen, you can use carob as a substitute in baking and desserts.

Eggs All fresh pasta is made with eggs, so if eggs are an allergen, never assume that spaghetti is safe. And be careful of cheese fillings, as in manicotti, that may also contain eggs.

Nuts Peanuts are not really nuts but are often allergens for people who react to nuts.

Shellfish If shellfish are allergens, you may or may not react to other fish.

Wheat   If wheat is an allergen, don't assume rye bread is safe. Rye bread usually contains more wheat than rye flour.

Yeast Not all baked goods are made with yeast, but many breads are. It's not hard to learn which are which. If yeast is an allergen for you, avoid foods that contain molds (see box Foods to Avoid If Molds Are an Allergen, page 172).

sensitive to the six sulfites used as preservatives—sulfur diozide, sodium sulfite, sodium and potassium bisulfite, and sodium and potassium metabisulfite." The FDA warns that although "industry representatives have said that sulfites are not commonly used on frozen potatoes, some apparently are treated. These treated products are required to have a declaration on their packages. However, a sulfite-sensitive person eating in a restaurant ordinarily would not see the label and thus might be at risk." (Most people are not sulfite-sensitive, which is one of the reasons a ban was so long in coming.)

If, during or shortly after eating, you experience nausea, diarrhea, hives, flushing, weakness, swollen tongue, or difficulty in swallowing or breathing, or feel faint, you may be sulfite-sensitive and should check with your doctor. Severe reactions of this sort require immediate emergency treatment (they also, of course, may be caused by allergies to substances other than sulfites or may be due to entirely different causes).

Unfortunately, if you are sensitive, you must also be alert in the emergency room, since sodium bisulfite is used as a preservative in epinephrine, which is routinely used for treating severe asthmatic reactions. It is puzzling that sulfites are permitted in a

---

How to Avoid Sulfites

If you want to know what foods contain sulfites, look at the label for bisulfite, potassium metabisulfite, sodium bisulfite, sodium sulfite, or sulfur diozide. Among the foods that may contain this additive are cookies and other bakery products (from the dough conditioner); raw, frozen, canned, and dehydrated potatoes (including french fries, cottage fries, and hash browns in restaurants); maraschino cherries; corn syrup; shellfish and other seafood (they are often sulfited on the fishing boats); salad dressings; pickles; wine and beer; dried fruits; and many processed foods, such as soups. In addition, surimi (don't think of it as just fish or pollock—it contains a lot of other things, including eggs) contains sulfites, so all imitation products made from it, including crabmeat, shrimp, lobster, and scallops, should be avoided.

number of prescription and nonprescription drugs used by asthmatics (including some used in nebulizers), and at present it is very much a case of let the buyer beware. If you have a neighborhood pharmacist who keeps information on your prescriptions on a computer, ask him to let you know if you receive any prescriptions that contain sulfites. If you can pick a time when he isn't too busy, ask him if it would be possible to get a list of all asthma drugs that contain sulfites so that you, too, can keep track.

Before the ban sulfites were commonly used in salad bar items, to prevent lettuce and other vegetables from browning and thus keep things looking fresh longer. Now, however, many restaurants have voluntarily discontinued their use and are more aware of what items contain them in case you should ask.

If you have a sulfite sensitivity, ask about it also when you purchase take-out food and deli items, including coleslaw, avocado dips, and cut-up fresh fruit.

Artificial Colors   There is no reason to expose yourself to any artificial colors and it is better to avoid foods that contain them when you can, but there is one that asthmatics who are sensitive to aspirin should take particular care to avoid; this is tartrazine, or yellow food dye #5. Over the years the FDA has made gestures toward banning it, but so far the only restriction is that it must be specifically listed on the label. So here again, read the label where there is one.

Restaurant food doesn't usually come labeled, but the other night the Chinese restaurant I was in brought the end-of-the-meal fortune cookies individually wrapped. I had never seen that before and idly read the tiny print on the wrapper: "Flour, Sugar, Water, Lecithin, Partially Hydrogenated Corn Oil, Eggs, FD Yellow #5 & #6. Artificial Flavoring, BHT, Salt." The moral is, always read labels when you have the chance (and if you have a reaction after eating fortune cookies, it may not mean you are allergic or sensitive to eggs).

Other Additives and Preservatives   It is impossible to avoid eating all food that contains additives and preservatives, but label reading will help you avoid a great many of them, such as artificial colors and artificial flavors. Given a choice of products, pick the one with the fewest ingredients. That way you will be more likely to get closer to food as nature originally intended it to be eaten, and to avoid all the modern "helpers" that your great-grand-mother managed to do without.

If you should have a reaction to a food, try to find out what is in it; it may be something added in the processing, rather than the food itself, that is causing the problem. Even fresh produce can cause a reaction, because of pesticides and insecticides on the peel and in the wax coating. Many supermarkets now sell fresh organic fruits and vegetables, so if you are very fond of a pro-cessed food that you think may be making you sick, ask your doctor whether you might try cooking an organic version of it from scratch at home yourself.

Ethnic Foods   Our eating has become much more cosmopolitan in recent years, which is fun, but this trend has made identifying specific allergens more difficult. Chinese food is a good example. A few years ago a reaction known as Chinese Restaurant Syn-drome made the news as more and more people reported un-pleasant facial symptoms, difficulty breathing, and headaches, after eating in Chinese restaurants. The cause was found to be monosodium glutamate (MSG), which most Chinese chefs rou-tinely added as a flavor enhancer. It is a very old and normally safe additive, except that a number of people appear to be sensi-tive to it.

Many Chinese restaurants no longer use it, and if they do and you ask that it be omitted when you order, almost all restaurants will leave it out. In the few dishes where this is not possible because it has already been incorporated in one or more ingredi-ents, the waiter will usually tell you.

Indonesian and Greek cuisines use eggs in many entrees, and sometimes unfamiliar spices will mask the taste of ingredients you usually avoid. Do not hesitate to try new foods, but notice if you have a reaction and perhaps avoid that particular food for a while, or at least until you can determine what ingredient in the dish you are reacting to. Even familiar foods eaten in a new restaurant need to be approached with some attention. For instance, if you are allergic to eggs, you may be baffled when a favorite Chinese dish that you have always eaten with impunity suddenly causes a reaction. The problem may be egg white, which is optional in many Chinese recipes; some chefs use it and some don't, especially in the sauces.

(Egg white can be found in many unexpected places; for example, it is sometimes used as a wash to create a shine on baked goods. You may notice, if you are allergic to eggs, that you can tell almost immediately when you put an egg-containing food in your mouth. Once you have identified this feeling, it will prevent you from swallowing the mouthful; you can then unobtrusively dispose of it in a napkin and get on with your meal.)

Molds   If mold seems to trigger your asthma, you will usually be advised to avoid foods that contain, or tend to quickly generate, molds. This could include anything made with yeast, such as bread, especially sour-dough types, and some cakes.

Fermented beverages and foods—wine, beer, sauerkraut, cider, and vinegar (as well as foods made with vinegar, such as salad dressings and condiments)—may bother you. Blue, Roquefort, and other mold cheeses are especially to be avoided, and all smoked seafood and meats (to be safe, just don't eat the usual delicatessen meats, except for roast beef and turkey), including frankfurters and many sausages. Be careful of foods refrigerated past their prime; try to date the packages if you tend to lose track, or just throw them out if you are doubtful.

Health Foods   The government does not define health foods or what may be so labeled, so there is no more jurisdiction over them than over other foods. If you are allergic or have food sensitivities or intolerances, the fact that a food is sold by a health food store will not make it any better for you; also, you may be intrigued by unfamiliar foods and try them without being as careful to read the labels as you would be in the supermarket.

If you are trying unfamiliar health foods, do so cautiously.

Foods to Avoid If Molds Are an Allergen

Baked goods made with yeast   Cookies and layer cakes are usually safe, but breads, Danish pastry, coffee cake, and other baked goods should be checked out before eating. If you're very sensitive to yeast, you may be able to detect it by breaking off a small piece and smelling it.

Buttermilk and sour cream

Cheeses   Especially Roquefort, Gorgonzola, Stilton, and similar cheeses.

Fermented and pickled products   These include vinegars, pickles, pickled vegetables (including sauerkraut), and soy sauce, among other items.

Mushrooms

Wine, beer, and other alcoholic beverages

Note: Do not eat foods that are old, even if they have been refrigerated. Learn to recognize mold and discard food that has become at all moldy. Do not just cut the mold off cheese, because it may have eaten deeper than you think. Theoretically, it is all right to take the mold off jelly and still use it, but a mold-sensitive person should not take any chances.

Even something that seems intrinsically harmless, such as herbal teas, may be hazardous to someone with allergies. For instance, camomile flowers make a soothing tea that is sometimes recommended as a soporific. Unfortunately, if you get hay fever or are allergic to pollens, you may be allergic to camomile. When eating or drinking something new, try to get it in its simplest form so that if you get a reaction, you don't have to puzzle out which of a long list of ingredients caused your problem.

Food/Drug Interactions

Many drugs are affected by foods as well as by climate and other extraneous factors. Doctors should tell you this, but even the best of them sometimes forget to or assume, if it's a common drug like tetracycline, that you already know. Happily, most pharmacists put this information on the label, along with the name of the drug and when it should be taken. To be absolutely safe, always ask the pharmacist when you pick up the prescription whether there is anything you should or shouldn't take it with. It's a good idea to keep a small book of personal medical information and to write this down as soon as you find out.

Drugs that are hard on the stomach, such as oral steroids, should be taken with food; even half a glass of milk is enough, so if it isn't convenient to coordinate your medication with meal-times, or if you forget to take it then, just sip some milk when you do take it. On the other hand, some drugs should definitely not be taken with milk; you may have to wait an hour or more after having milk or dairy products before you take them.

The effect of taking theophylline with food seems to vary; some people on high doses experience an enhanced effect, which is especially undesirable if you are already on a high dose, so it is important to check with your doctor. Also ask what he or she considers "food." A glass of whole milk, with its high fat content, or a bowl of buttered popcorn may be enough to cause a problem. (See also pages 35–45.)

In general, it's best to swallow tablets and capsules with plain water. Some people reach for whatever liquid is handy (orange juice, club soda, cider, coffee, beer), but this is not a good idea because some liquids increase the action of certain drugs and some counteract it to such an extent that you may get the effect of only a small part of the prescribed dose. As we have seen, coffee and some other beverages, such as colas, are liable to increase the action of theophylline (which is closely related to caffeine), and since the safety margin of theophylline is somewhat narrow, this could be serious (see box, page 37).

The Bottom Line

Given the dearth of definitive knowledge as to what sort of diet would most benefit an asthmatic, and the confusion and contro-versy over which foods are healthful, and which are not, how can the consumer know what constitutes a balanced, healthful diet?

The answer is, you can't really *know* but you can make an educated guess.

The best advice has actually not changed from what it was decades ago: eat a wide variety of foods and eat them with as little processing as possible. The wide variety will in itself ensure better nutrition because you will get the different nutrients available in the different foods; for instance, eating vegetables of all colors—green, red, orange, beige—and all types, from salad greens to root vegetables, will automatically provide a good range of vitamins and minerals. Eat them as much in season as possible.

Do not be fooled by availability into thinking something is in season. Thanks to modern distribution methods, most fruits and vegetables are available in our supermarkets throughout the year—sometimes shipped from countries as far away as Australia. Remember, even fresh produce from California has to travel three thousand miles to get to the East Coast. If you can buy produce grown locally, so much the better.

Out-of-season produce may be less nutritious than frozen, so when fresh fruits and vegetables are especially expensive, it's fairly safe to assume they are out of season, and it might be more nutritious to switch to frozen. Sometimes even canned vegetables are more nutritious than out-of-season fresh—whole canned tomatoes, for example.

Again, eat as few processed foods as possible and choose the least processed—plain regular oatmeal, for example, over flavored (add your own sprinkle of cinnamon) and enriched. Save money and take vitamin supplements out of your own medicine chest instead of buying foods expensively bolstered with them.

Go easy on sugar (learn all its names, such as corn syrup, so you can recognize oversugared foods, such as cereal that depends on added sugars for its flavor), and try to keep fat consumption down to the 30 percent mark.

Don't fall for food fads. When a new study seems to indicate, for instance, that certain high-fiber foods are good for you, or that eggs are bad, pay attention to any experts who don't agree. They have less of an ax to grind and are often the voice of reason in a world of hype. Anyhow, if you are eating a wide variety of foods, you are probably getting sufficient fiber, and the fiber needed by the human body is not just one kind but a number of kinds. And as for eggs, notice the official wording on foods labeled "No Cholesterol." It reads: "Information on fat and cholesterol is provided for individuals who, on the advice of a physician, are modifying their total dietary intake of fat and/or cholesterol." If it had really been proved that cholesterol was unhealthy for healthy people, the government would not require the manufacturer to take up precious label space with this hedge.

The trend is to simpler foods—natural juices instead of heavy syrups for canned fruit, less fat in everything, a return to basics. This is a good time to start eating right, so go with it.

Part Four

Asthma and Exercise

16

Exercise and
Your Respiratory System

When I first started to work with a respiratory rehabilitation therapist, one of the words I heard most often as the reason for problems I was encountering was "deconditioning"—the reduction of physical strength and stamina. Did I have a problem climbing stairs? "Deconditioning." Did I need to stroll instead of walking briskly? "Deconditioning." Did I have to rest in between swimming laps? "Deconditioning." I soon realized that what I was really being told was that it wasn't my asthma that was holding me back but my poor physical condition, and that I would feel better when I was fitter. This was the first inkling I had that something other than drugs and avoiding triggers could help my asthma.

At the time I didn't realize that an additional point was being made: not all my breathing problems and poor stamina were due to asthma. Anyone with a chronic disease falls into the habit of ascribing everything, from ordinary tiredness to normal everyday complaints, to the disease. We forget there are only a few symptoms to go around, and any given one may be caused by a number of different factors. Once you realize this, you will not only be a better diagnostician, you will also feel less limited by your asthma; it may not be nearly as pervasive as you have been thinking.

Obesity

It is undesirable to be out of shape, but if you are also obese, that compounds the problem. Carrying around a lot of extra weight is hard on your whole system and obviously makes asthma more difficult because of the increased amount of oxygen needed. Happily, slimming down will be beneficial in a number of ways, so think of the additional difficulty being overweight causes your asthma as further motivation to get in shape.

What If Exercising Gets Me Out of Breath?

There is a natural tendency among people with asthma to exercise less and less. The thought of bringing on an asthma attack is enough to make anyone think twice about an activity, and if exercise seems to make breathing more difficult, it is only natural to cut back. After all, we know exercise is the trigger for exercise-induced asthma, and we also know that running, walking briskly, and similar activities make even nonasthmatics breathe harder, so it would seem that asthmatics are better off taking it easy. Mothers with asthmatic children tend to caution them against running, going out for sports, and indulging in other strenuous activities, and most adults think asthma and athletics are incompatible. This is an unfortunate misconception; just the opposite is true.

A certain amount of shortness of breath with great exertion is normal for everyone; the greater the exertion, the greater the shortness of breath. Marathon and Olympic runners expect to reach the finish line out of breath, and it takes a while for even these trained runners to breathe comfortably again. On the other hand, many people with asthma appear to react badly to even a low level of activity; someone with asthma can get out of breath climbing a short flight of stairs.

Getting out of breath with minor exertion is not normal, even in most cases of asthma. If you have been having this problem, good management plus rehabilitation through an individually designed exercise program and training in breathing exercises will bear out the attitude of Dr. Charles Reed of the Mayo Clinic, who says, "Most people with asthma don't need to be disabled, impaired, or even restricted now."

Since an optimistic attitude is important, start by not blaming all your breathing problems on the severity of your asthma; you may be selling yourself short and denying yourself activities unnecessarily. Of course, your condition needs to be evaluated by a professional, and before you embark on any sort of physical conditioning or exercise program, check with your doctor or respiratory rehab therapist. The therapist will plan an individual program geared to your actual condition and the seriousness of your asthma. If the best you can do in the beginning is exercise while sitting in a chair, that's no problem; if you have the will, your therapist will show you the way.

Why Is It Particularly Important for an Asthmatic to Be Fit?

Between symptoms you probably show no signs of asthma and appear perfectly "normal." Theoretically, if you could avoid all asthma triggers or reduce your twitchy airway reactions, you would never have another attack. Since asthma is not considered curable, that is unlikely to happen. It is, however, reversible, which means that the better your physical condition, the better the disease.

There is even some evidence that exercise may reduce the degree of the reactivity of the airways. Exercise-induced asthma, for instance, has the peculiar characteristic of sometimes responding to a long warm-up (twenty minutes, for instance) with reduced airway reactivity. If someone with EIA warms up that way shortly before strenuous exercise, he or she may find that the EIA doesn't occur. Jackie Joyner-Kersee, an Olympic champion, uses this system. She finds, however, that if too long a time elapses between warm-up and exertion, the inhibitory effect wears off. It's as if the mediator-releasing mast cells that trigger bronchospasm have had time to recharge and are ready to act again. The mast-cell reaction almost seems to function like the automatic flash on a camera; if you use the flash and then pause to give it time to recharge, it is ready to function again. (For a full discussion of techniques of coping with EIA, see Chapter 18.)

In addition to contributing to general good health, exercise will benefit your asthma through the strengthening of certain specific physical areas. Your respiratory muscles are a good example of how being fit will help your body cope.

Respiratory Muscles (see also Chapter 17)

When breathing is not a problem, we don't realize how many muscles are directly involved in that simple, essential action. There are three different sets of muscles used for normal breathing.

1. The *diaphragm* is a dome-shaped muscle situated horizontally between the chest and the abdomen. It is the primary breathing muscle and does up to 80 percent of the work of breathing.

When you breathe in, the diaphragm flattens out, contracting downward and making room for more air in your lungs. When you breathe out, it relaxes, expanding upward and decreasing the air space to help you expel the air. By learning diaphragmatic breathing (see next chapter), you strengthen this key muscle and help it to work more efficiently.

2. The *intercostal muscles* are found between the ribs and control the movement of the ribs. There are two different kinds: the external and the internal.

When you breathe in, the external intercostal muscles increase lung capacity by contracting and pulling the ribs up and outward. When you breathe out, the internal intercostal muscles reverse the process, helping to expel the air. If you put your hands on either side of your rib cage, you can feel your ribs expand and contract as these muscles do their job.

3. The *accessory breathing muscles* play a secondary role, primarily during greater exertion than that created by ordinary breathing.

The large abdominal muscles help in breathing out; they are used when you speak or sing and also for the explosive air flow of a sneeze or a cough. Diaphragmatic breathing exercises help strengthen these muscles, and teach you how to use them for increased physical activity.

Neck, shoulder, and back muscles are sometimes called on when the other breathing muscles are not getting enough oxygen into the system. If you notice your shoulders have become hunched and your neck is getting stiff, you are probably trying to breathe with these muscles. Unfortunately, they are not particularly efficient helpers, and the sooner you can relax your shoulders and go back to using the main breathing muscles, the sooner you will get control of your breathing. Relaxation techniques can help you make this transition, but it takes a great deal of control and conscious effort to try to relax when asthma is severe. If relaxation techniques are a regular part of your daily routine, it will be much easier to call on them in a time of stress.

Some asthmatics have gotten so in the habit of using these muscles that their posture and body shape are affected; hunched, rounded shoulders and a barrel chest are characteristic of long-term improper breathing. The diaphragm may have become weaker because of poor utilization and will need to be strengthened gradually. Obviously, it is better to learn to breathe correctly before this happens.

The Heart

Many people with asthma worry about the strain it may be putting on their hearts. Although this is not generally the case, a healthy heart (also a muscle) is certainly desirable. The important role regular exercise plays in keeping the heart healthy is well documented, and aerobic exercise has become a national pastime. But in the beginning exercise doesn't have to be aerobic to be helpful. Today postoperative patients—even after bypass surgery—are gotten out of bed and on their feet in a matter of days, and mild, gentle exercise is started almost immediately. Cardiovascular exercise is now considered an essential part of any exercise regime, and the level can be tailored to your own individual limitations.

Asthmatics are fortunate that they can participate in all of the best heart-healthy exercises, such as walking and swimming; with perseverance athletes with asthma have found they can compete in almost any sport that gives them pleasure. Do get professional evaluation before you start. A respiratory therapist will see that a person who has been sedentary works up to real exertion at a slower pace than someone who is already walking three miles every morning. Effective training also requires knowing when to increase the pace and duration of a given exercise so that it is a challenge without being a strain.

The Immune System

Since asthma has been ascribed to an overactive immune system because of the immune system's reaction to "triggers," it would be helpful to tell you what to do to make it less reactive. This is an area in which intensive research is being done all over the world, and it is the basis of preventive treatment, such as prescribing inhaled steroids to reduce the incidence of inflammation.

There are some clues as to what may lead to a healthier immune system. Exercise not only improves your general health but, as we have discussed, helps you to deal with stress—which is now thought to lower immunity—and also to have a better self-image and maintain a more positive outlook.

We have said that exercise won't cure asthma, because there are no studies showing that this has ever happened. But exercise has been shown to increase lung capacity, and any asthmatic will consider this a worthy achievement. There is also no doubt that feeling fit increases self-confidence and a feeling of control, which carries over to personal asthma management. Feelings of anxiety, panic, and being out of control are less likely to occur when you are fit than when you are already physically and emotionally debilitated.

How Much Exercise?

To be beneficial, exercise must be done regularly. Vacations with a nonstop round of activity for two or three weeks a year or weekend golf and tennis games won't do the job. Present guidelines recommend a minimum of twenty minutes of aerobic exercise (and there are many kinds of aerobic exercise besides the bouncing-up-and-down kind we see on TV) about three times a week for a "normal" person. But everyone, with or without asthma, has to work up his or her own fitness schedule. An individualized exercise program, supervised by a therapist, is the best way for an asthmatic to achieve maximum fitness.

Getting Started

1. *Don't start on your own.* Talk with your doctor. If you don't have a respiratory therapist, this is a good time to get one.

2. *Gauge how you're feeling before you start.* If you are having trouble breathing, do what you can to get comfortable (use your inhaler about twenty minutes before you start, for instance). I like to start out with a slow walk, especially if it's the first exercise of the day, and then proceed to whatever exercise I want to do.

If your breathing worsens with exercise, stop and rest until you are in control again. Your doctor and your therapist can give you tips on how to handle yourself under various conditions and when it may be a good idea to take the day off or postpone exercise until later.

If you can't exercise that day, try to keep as active as possible. Do little chores and rest frequently if necessary. Inactivity can by itself make your breathing worse. For instance, if you sit quietly reading for an hour or two, you may find that merely getting up to make a cup of tea makes you breathe harder. This kind of breathlessness often improves if you just move around slowly and get yourself going again.

3. *Think of all activity as exercise.* There are many everyday things you do that can be altered slightly so they become exercise. For example, if you drive to the market, park farther away than usual so you have to walk a little more to get to the market. If your house or apartment has stairs, use them, as slowly as necessary and faster when you can. (One of the most popular machines in health clubs simulates stair climbing.)

4. *Prepare yourself.* Choose a time of day when you usually feel best and are not already overtired. Take your medicine on schedule and follow the doctor's instructions for extra medication before exertion. Dress for your exercise (loose, comfortable clothing, suitable footwear). If it is part of a daily routine, try to do it at the same time every day so that it becomes as automatic as brushing your teeth.

5. *Stretch before you start.* Animals know enough to do this, but people aren't always so smart. A cat will stretch each and every time it gets up, even if it has been sitting only a little while—and not many animals keep themselves as fit as a cat. Stretching feels good and requires very little breath, so you can stretch even on the days when nothing more strenuous feels good. It's an especially good idea to stretch for a few minutes in bed before getting up in the morning.

When watching TV, reading, or doing anything that could keep you sitting for long periods of time, break your activity briefly and do a few stretching exercises. If you can, stand up and walk around for a minute or two while doing them. Since most people don't drink enough liquids, you can also use this time to get a drink of water or juice.

6. *Always warm up and cool down.* Even professionals begin slowly and end up slowly. If you watch sports on TV, notice how the athletes warm up (baseball pitchers even have a special place where they can do this). This gives your body, especially your heart and muscles, a chance to adjust to a higher level of activity. It minimizes strain and is the only beneficial way to exercise.

7. *Start slowly and work up gradually.* Starting is easy; just start out by being more active than you were yesterday. If you spent five minutes outdoors yesterday, spend ten today. If you walked a mile, walk a mile and a quarter, or increase your pace a little. Stay with your new goal until it feels easy and automatic; then increase slowly again. Each time your body has adjusted to the new goal, stretch it a little by doing a little more. Never exercise to the point of real fatigue; it should always feel good.

Don't use bad weather as an excuse not to exercise. In the following pages are many exercises to do indoors, and you don't need fancy exercise equipment to do them (although equipment can be fun and often makes it easier to follow a regime).

8. *"But exercise is boring."* It needn't be. Boring is a state of mind; being sick is much more boring than exercise, so work on finding ways to make your exercise periods interesting. Concentrate on how good it feels to be doing something instead of sitting around. Take a look in the mirror after you've reached the point of doing real serious exercise and working up a sweat; your skin will glisten and look rosy, your eyes will sparkle, and sometimes even some of those small wrinkles you've been noticing will seem less visible.

There are many ways to add interest to exercises. For instance, riding a stationary bike can get monotonous, but I do it with the TV on. This worked fine except on Saturday mornings when most of the programs are kiddie cartoons. Then I discovered that some of the cartoons weren't bad, and now I have my favorites and sometimes bike much longer than I am supposed to because I want to see the rest of the program; the time just flies. There are even book rests that enable you to read or study while biking.

Later on in Part Four you will find more tips for keeping your interest up while exercising.

The Best Types of Exercise for Asthmatics

Stop-and-Go Sports   Tennis, bowling, and golf are nonaerobic sports and are not rated as heart-healthy exercises because they do not require sustained effort, but that is exactly why they work for asthmatics. The break in activity, waiting for the ball to come back over the net or for your partner to take a turn, gives you a chance to catch your breath.

Sustained, team activity that requires you to keep up other players' pace is often not the best choice because you are likely to do more than is good for you and to feel embarrassed if you have to drop out or fall behind. On the other hand, if there is a sport you especially like to play, give it a try. With proper premedication and a good warm-up, you may be able to do more than you think. After all, there are athletes with asthma playing in just about every professional sport. Any generalization as to what sports someone with asthma can participate in successfully is subject to exceptions. Cross-country skiing, one of the most strenuous of all sports and one done in a cold environment, can be enjoyed by many people with asthma. Be sensible, but be persistent if there is something you particularly want to do. And always work with a pulmonary professional until you have mastered the self-care it involves.

Diaphragmatic and Pursed-Lip Breathing   All asthmatics, regardless of their activity level, will do better when they learn how to breathe. You may think you already know how (after all, you can prove you are breathing), but if you are not familiar with these breathing exercises and don't practice them regularly, you are depriving yourself of one of the easiest ways to improve and control your asthma. The next chapter will show you how to do them.

17

Pursed-Lip and Diaphragmatic Breathing

Most people don't pay much attention to their breathing, but people with asthma, especially if it is not under control or if they are deconditioned, may not have enough breath to walk comfortably up a flight of stairs. And many more asthmatics, who have no problem with everyday activities that don't make any real demands on their lung capacity, have difficulty finding enough breath to do aerobics, go for a brisk walk (especially uphill), go cross-country skiing, or engage in sex. If this is your problem, you may not be breathing as efficiently as you can.

A certain amount of shortness of breath with exertion is normal, but you can tell if you get out of breath more quickly than most people. If you do, breathing retraining may help you breathe more like everyone else.

There are three breathing exercises that anyone with asthma should learn and practice regularly: pursed-lip breathing, diaphragmatic breathing, and advanced diaphragmatic breathing.

Pursed-lip breathing is usually done in conjunction with one of the other two breathing exercises, although it can be done alone.

Pursed-Lip Breathing

How to Do It

1. Close your mouth and inhale through your nose. (If your nose is too stuffed, breathe through your mouth slowly.)

2. Purse your lips (as if about to whistle or blow out a candle) and exhale slowly through your mouth. *Do not blow out hard;* use as little force as possible to keep exhaling.

3. Count as you exhale; exhale twice as long as you inhale. For instance, inhale for a count of two; exhale for a count of four. (To keep from counting too fast, try saying to yourself "one thousand and one, one thousand and two," and so on.) If you can't do it for that long, do the best you can. You should find you can increase the count a little as your breathing becomes more efficient.

Since exhaling is more difficult for an asthmatic than inhaling, try to breathe out the best you can. Don't, however, feel you should be expelling every little bit of breath in your lungs; that wouldn't be a good idea even if you could do it (you can't).

In the beginning it will take a lot of concentration, but it's a very helpful way to breathe and can be used to relax and to slow your breathing down when you are short of breath and breathing faster and shallower. It will also help provide breath for all kinds of exercises; if you watch sports, you will find athletes doing it after an especially strenuous event.

What Not to Do

1. Again, don't breathe out hard. I've read books and articles that say you should breathe out hard enough so the air comes out almost with a hiss or a whistle, but no doctor or rehab respiratory nurse/therapist I've ever interviewed agrees with this. Hard, forced exhalation is liable to cause your airway muscles to constrict.

Breathe out slowly and gently, staying as relaxed as possible. Some therapists advise letting the exhaled air sort of dribble out naturally through pursed lips, but I find a little bit of pressure works best for me.

2. Don't hold your breath between breathing in and breathing out.

3. Stop doing it if it makes you feel light-headed or dizzy.

When and Where to Do Pursed-Lip Breathing

As noted above, this exercise can be used to slow down your breathing when you are tense or short of breath and to provide more breath when you exercise. It is helpful:

1. when your breathing is getting more rapid than normal.
2. when you're feeling anxious.
3. when you feel a little out of breath.
4. when you're doing diaphragmatic breathing.
5. when exercising. The general rule is to inhale before exertion, exhale during exertion.
6. when you're waiting to see the doctor.
7. when you're feeling very stressed.
8. when you notice your neck and shoulder muscles getting tight. In this case, gently try the exercises, such as shoulder rolls (see pages 211–12), that relax these muscles.
9. any other time when you feel it might help.

Some instructions suggest, when you are first learning, that you start when lying down on a bed or the floor, but if you are having trouble breathing, this may not be the most comfortable position. It is best to be as comfortable and as relaxed as possible, although you can do pursed-lip breathing anywhere in almost any position.

In the beginning I found it best to start while sitting in a straight chair. Then try doing it while walking around. Eventually, you will probably find you can do it lying down, driving a car, or wherever you need to. If you're in a public place, you can do it fairly unobtrusively, and unless you are looking directly at someone, no one will even notice.

Practice it several times a day until it becomes second nature to breathe that way when you need help or are doing anything that makes you breathless (if you run for a bus or climb stairs too quickly, it's a pleasant and easy way to regain control).

Do it with your morning exercises (ask your therapist if you aren't able to figure out at what point to breathe in or exhale with a particular exercise), or just do it by itself daily to continue to improve your breathing efficiency and as a relaxation technique.

Diaphragmatic Breathing

Although diaphragmatic breathing by itself is useful in some professions—for instance, playing a wind instrument, singing in opera—and on other occasions where breath control is important, it is helpful for someone with asthma, especially when combined with pursed-lip breathing.

Diaphragmatic breathing accomplishes three things:

1. *Slower, deeper breathing* is inevitable when you do diaphragmatic breathing. When you are having trouble breathing, you tend to almost pant in an effort to get air into your lungs more quickly. This has the opposite effect and usually makes matters worse. This combination will help you regain control.

2. *Improved lung function* is achieved. Because this technique uses the diaphragm, the main breathing muscle, it strengthens it and makes it more efficient. With improper breathing the diaphragm may not get enough use and may lose strength and elasticity.

3. *Relaxation* is enhanced. Just having something to do at a time when your asthma is acting up is in itself relaxing and leads to less anxiety. In addition, as your combination breathing becomes slower and deeper it will become more efficient, with a greater amount of air moving in and out of the lungs, so that you are breathing more normally and providing your body with more oxygen; you cannot help but relax as you realize you are actually managing your asthma. When you are having an attack, it will not take the place of necessary medication, but relaxing will help the medication do its job.

How to Do Diaphragmatic Breathing

Lie down, or stand or sit in front of a mirror, with one hand on your stomach, the other on your chest. (If you lie down, bend your knees and put a pillow behind them.) Relax your stomach, chest, and shoulder muscles.

Now take a deep breath through your nose. If the hand on your chest moves while the hand on your stomach doesn't budge, you are not breathing efficiently and you are not breathing from your diaphragm. Breathe out through your mouth, and concentrate on keeping your chest from moving.

Your stomach should rise under your hand each time as you breathe in, then deflate and flatten as you breathe out; it's all right to help by gradually pulling in your stomach muscles when you breathe out.

When you have successfully done that a few times, add pursed-lip breathing (see pages 190–92). In other words, breathe in through your nose so that your abdomen, not your chest, expands. Then, without a pause, breathe out from your abdomen with the pursed-lip breathing technique. Keep your muscles as relaxed as possible when performing this exercise.

The important next step is to do it while walking around, and once you have mastered that, you can do it anytime: exercising, watching TV, working, or doing chores.

In the beginning breathe in and out about ten times and return to your normal breathing pattern. Gradually increase the exercise period until you are doing it about twenty minutes a day. Your doctor or rehab respiratory nurse/therapist will be able to help you master this technique and check that you are doing it correctly. The therapist will also explain how to apply the technique to ordinary, everyday activities, such as climbing stairs, reaching high shelves, having sex, or doing your daily calisthenics. If you have been getting out of breath performing simple, routine tasks, you will be pleasantly surprised at how much easier they suddenly are to do.

Advanced Diaphragmatic Breathing

Once you have learned regular diaphragmatic breathing, you may want to advance to *lower rib expansion.* With this exercise you expand your lower ribs rather than your abdomen. It makes your breathing even more efficient, will expand your lower chest, and is good for the tone of your diaphragm.

How to Do It

Sit in a chair and put your hands on the sides of your lower ribs (slightly higher than your navel but on either side of your body). Follow the same instructions as for regular diaphragmatic breathing, but expand and contract your lower ribs instead of your abdomen. Still keeping your chest from moving, try to breathe so that you can feel your sides (sort of the top of your abdomen) expand. This is a little tricky; at first you will probably just expand your abdomen, and when you try not to do that, you will tend to breathe with your chest. Persevere, and after a couple of tries you will suddenly find the right spot expanding. Your abdomen will still expand somewhat, but you will know you are doing it right because the hands on your lower ribs will move as you breathe in and out.

To check, try a few breaths from your abdomen with your hands on your lower ribs, and you will see that your hands don't move at all even when your abdomen is visibly expanding and contracting.

I find that rib expansion is easier to keep track of if I place my thumb a little more to the back and the rest of my hand facing front (the way a cross person stands with hands on hips—only a little higher), but your pulmonary rehab nurse/therapist may have other tips to help you master this exercise.

The Next Step

Now you've learned how to control your breathing; improve your lung capacity; strengthen your primary breathing muscle, the diaphragm; relax; and enlarge your range of activities and ease of doing them. The next step is to see what kind of regular exercise will work best with the limitations you may encounter because of asthma. Everyone needs regular exercise to stay well; in some ways, as we have found, asthmatics need it even more than people without a chronic breathing disorder, but every case of asthma is different, so you need to discover what will work best for you.

Note: Not all pulmonary specialists agree that exercise will improve your pulmonary function, but asthmatics who have gone the exercise route seem to find that it works. Nancy Hogshead, in her book *Asthma and Exercise* says, "My asthma seems to get worse whenever I begin to lose my physical conditioning." I myself definitely notice the difference in my asthma if I am inactive for any length of time, and conversely, the more active I am, the less medication I seem to need.

Even physicians who are not convinced of the value of these "breathing exercises" conceded that exercise of any kind improves your overall health, builds cardiopulmonary fitness, improves circulation, and tends to foster a more optimistic and cheerful frame of mind. And they tend to agree that all exercise has a favorable effect on the immune system. In sum, even those doctors who weren't exercise enthusiasts where asthma was concerned agreed that it might indirectly have a beneficial effect. I have found from my own experience that it certainly does; why not give breathing exercises a try and see if they work for you?

18

The Truth About
Asthma and Exercise

Years ago it was thought that asthma and exercise didn't mix. To some extent that myth still persists, but we now know that asthmatics can and should exercise. Regular exercise not only contributes to good health but may decrease the incidence of heart disease, reduce obesity and serum cholesterol, and increase longevity. For someone with asthma, one of the most important benefits of exercise—in addition to being an enjoyable part of a normal life—is that it can increase breathing capacity and improve lung function. If you like sports but have ben afraid that participating might bring on an asthma attack, you will be glad to hear that you can learn to manage your asthma so that you can enjoy physical activity free from fear.

Because not being able to breathe can be so frightening, an asthmatic who has found that exercising seems to trigger symptoms is bound to cut back. This creates a vicious circle; the less you exercise, the more easily you will get out of breath, until just getting up to get a glass of water may make you breathless.

Each person's asthma is unique, and the degree of activity possible varies with the individual; one person may be able to be a professional athlete while another may be more limited. Your doctor or respiratory nurse/therapist can evaluate your potential activity level and help you reach it. If you try to do this on your own, you are liable either to do less than you can and never discover what you are really capable of, or to start out too fast, become discouraged, and fall back to being comparatively inactive.

Exercise-induced Asthma (EIA) and Exercise-induced Bronchospasm (EIB)

It is true that exercise is in itself a common trigger for most people with asthma; this is reflected in the name exercise-induced asthma, or EIA (and exercise-induced bronchospasm, or EIB). Some people get only EIA and never have asthma at any other time. Others react to many triggers of which exercise is only one. Like other asthma triggers, EIA is reversible, and once you learn to manage it, you may find you can participate in sports, calisthenics, and similar activities to your heart's content. If you have any doubts on this score, perhaps it will give you confidence to know that many medal-winning Olympic athletes, such as Jackie Joyner-Kersee and Nancy Hogshead, have EIA.

What You Need to Know About EIA

It is thought that most people with asthma have EIA, but it is hard to measure the incidence of this problem because it often goes undiagnosed. This is because it is normal for strenuous exercise to cause some shortness of breath; thus EIA symptoms may not be recognized as anything special. If you have asthma and soon after starting a strenuous activity (running or swimming, for instance) begin to have difficulty breathing, become uncomfortably

---

Olympic Medal Winners with Asthma

When we read about famous athletes who are successful in their fields, we often have no way of knowing what obstacles they encountered on their way up. We tend to think of them as exceptionally talented, lucky, and usually above all, healthy. And sometimes we may think that if only we didn't have asthma, we, too, could do a lot better. If you have ever felt that way, here are some surprising facts.

The American Academy of Allergy and Immunology prepared a questionnaire for the members of the 1984 U.S. Summer Olympic team. Their answers indicated that 67 of the 597 members of the team had asthma, with symptoms of EIA or EIB. These 67 asthmatic Olympic athletes won 41 medals (out of a total of 174)—15 gold, 21 silver, and 5 bronze—in fourteen different events ranging from basketball to yachting. The greatest number of gold medals were the 5 in swimming, with 4 in basketball a close second. The greatest number of medals overall in any one category were 8 in cycling.

---

short of breath, start coughing, or feel very tight in your chest, you can assume you probably have EIA.

Although there are a number of theories, the physiological action that causes EIA is not clearly understood, but it has been shown that premedication before exercising can generally prevent it from developing. Your doctor will help determine the combination of medications that works best for you. The ones you take to premedicate before exertion may be an extension of those already prescribed for daily management of your asthma. For instance, if you already use an albuterol or terbutaline inhaler, you may add an extra premedication dose to your regular schedule. Cromolyn sodium, which has a different action and which some doctors prefer, is another possibility.

EIA takes several different forms. Sometimes asthma symptoms occur five to ten minutes into vigorous exercise but subside by themselves fairly quickly if you stop exercising for a short time.

With another form it is possible to work through mild EIA symptoms with a warm-up; in other words, continuing to exercise

Champion Athletes with Asthma

All the athletes listed here have asthma; they have reached the top in spite of it through good professional help from physicians, pulmonary rehab nurse/therapists, and coaches and, last but hardly least, through knowledgeable self-care. And though this list of champions is long, it barely scratches the surface of the numerous top athletes who have not let asthma hold them back.

Keith Brantley, runner. Among other honors, he was the Athletics Congress 1987 Road Racer of the Year. He has extrinsic asthma, and among his allergic triggers is tobacco smoke, to which he is so extremely sensitive that he claims he can tell when a car that passes him when he is running contains a passenger who is smoking.

Joe Carabino, basketball champion. All Ivy League, the European League.

Bruce Davidson, equestrian. A member of the Olympic equestrian team in 1972, 1976, 1984, and 1988, he was a medal winner in 1972 (silver team medal), 1976 (gold team medal), and 1984 (gold team medal). He is also the only person to date to win the world championship in individual Olympic equestrian competition twice (1974 and 1978), and he has been the American champion seven times so far. The most interesting fact of all about Bruce Davidson's asthma is that since childhood he has been allergic to horses.

Shirley Dery-Batlik, boating. She was a member of the 1984 U.S. Olympic canoeing and kayaking team.

Anita DeFrantz, rowing. She won a bronze medal in the 1976 Olympics in spite of her asthma, which she has had since childhood.

Rick DeMont, swimmer. He won a gold medal in the 1972 Olympics at the age of sixteen but never received it because he was disqualified when urine tests revealed ephedrine (from his Marax asthma medication), which through an oversight had not been cleared with the Olympic authorities.

Virginia Gilder, rowing. She won a silver team medal in the 1984 Olympics.

Mike Gminski, basketball. He is a center for the Philadelphia 76ers.

Alexi Grewal, cyclist. He won a gold medal in the 1984 Olympics. He tries to manage his extrinsic EIB with a nonpharmacological approach, which includes two-hour warm-ups, meditation, and special breathing techniques.

Nancy Hogshead, swimmer. In the 1984 Olympics she won a gold medal and the most medals overall won by any of the swimmers. Although she had EIA, she didn't know it until she had been swimming in competition for years, sometimes blacking out from lack of breath. Once diagnosed, she learned breathing and pacing techniques, went on to win Olympic medals, and today is such an enthusiastic supporter of exercise for asthmatics that she has written a book, *Asthma and Exercise.*

Jackie Joyner-Kersee, runner. Winner of two Olympic gold medals in 1988, she is currently the top-ranking track-and-field woman athlete.

Bill Koch, skier. He won a silver medal in the 1976 Olympics and the Cross-Country World Cup in 1982 and was a member of the 1984 Olympic team. His asthma was diagnosed in 1974.

Greg Louganis, diver. So far he has won four Olympic gold medals—two in the games at Los Angeles in 1984 and two in the 1988 games.

John Powell, discus thrower. He won Olympic bronze medals in 1976 and 1984 and has been a member of the last four Olympic teams (1972–88). Among his numerous achievements is his throw of 2265 feet, 8 inches, which set a world record in 1975; he was U.S. national champion in 1974, 1975, and 1983–87. His health problems were at first ascribed to allergies, and his asthma wasn't actually diagnosed until 1985.

Bonnie Warner, luge. She competed in the 1984 and 1988 Olympics as a member of the U.S. luge team. She has had asthma since childhood, and one of her main triggers is cold weather. (In case you don't know what luge is, it's a sledding sport that requires very cold weather conditions.)

causes the symptoms to subside, and it is then possible to proceed without further difficulty. The secret is to start exercising slowly; it won't work if you start out in high gear. It works so well for me that I tend to use mild exercise as a way to stop asthma symptoms if I notice when they are first coming on. I just get up and take a walk. (Of course, I don't hesitate to use my inhaler before starting out if I feel I need to.)

A third form of EIA does not manifest itself during the actual exercise but reaches its peak within five to ten minutes after you have stopped and, if not medicated, lasts from half an hour to an hour and a half before subsiding. Symptoms of this delayed reaction vary and may be breathlessness or coughing without wheezing. They are easy to recognize as EIA because the symptoms begin and continue long after nonasthmatics have gotten their breath back. It is typical of EIA that it tends to subside even without medication and rarely requires drastic measures.

It is possible to have different EIA reactions at different times or to sometimes exercise without having any of them (although if you are in competition, you wouldn't want to take the chance).

There is also some evidence that after an initial episode of EIA, subsequent occurrences may be milder, provided not too much time elapses between the EIA episode and the next exertion, although this is not invariable. Recent studies would appear to confirm this, and EIA is in fact described in an editorial in the August 30, 1987, issue of the *New England Journal of Medicine* as "self-limiting, spontaneously remitting, nonrecurrent airway narrowing in the majority."

EIA Trigger Enhancers

As the name indicates, the main trigger for EIA is exercise, but other factors may exacerbate the reactivity of the airways. If you are aware of these factors, you may wish to avoid exercising when they are present or take other protective measures, such as wearing a mask. You may be more liable to get EIA when you are not feeling up to scratch (maybe you are getting a cold and don't know it yet). Try to determine the cause when your reaction is out of the ordinary, but use your judgment as to whether to continue exercising.

Factors that may influence episodes of EIA include the following:

1. *The level of physical activity.* The more vigorous and sustained the activity, the greater the possibility of EIA.

2. *The degree of sensitivity of your airways.* This can vary from day to day and can be affected by external factors.

3. *Weather conditions.* Cold or very dry air is not as good an exercise environment as warm, humid air. When you know this, it is obvious why swimming is more likely to be a successful activity than skiing. You may find, however, that you personally can easily do both once you are conditioned, so do not rule out any sport unless your doctor or rehab nurse/therapist or your personal experience indicates you must, at least for the present.

4. *Altitude.* Unless conditioned to it, everyone has some difficulty adjusting to breathing and being active in high altitudes; even just strolling around can cause distress initially. If you are planning a trip to a place like Mexico City, you might want to talk to your doctor about managing asthma under these conditions. (Since Mexico City is also very polluted, it presents a double whammy for the asthmatic traveler and definitely calls for pre-planning.)

5. *Pollution* can exacerbate airway sensitivity whenever it occurs. Under this heading fall a number of things you may encounter unwittingly. For instance, air travel is frequently difficult because the air in the plane is extremely dry and, since it is recirculated, liable to be polluted. Fortunately, smoking has been banned by a number of airlines, but there are still many that permit it. European travel—in all forms of transportation, in restaurants, and at recreational events—will expose you to cigarette smoking above anything you have recently experienced in the United States, and as we have noted, you will be very much in the minority if you try to object to it.

If you have been sitting for a particularly long time in polluted air (a plane or a restaurant, for example), and get up quickly to walk, the sudden activity, with its increased oxygen demand, especially if you are hurrying, may cause breathlessness. I notice this after a transatlantic flight, when I have the long walk from the plane to the airport proper and am in a hurry to get where I am going. It is most liable to cause a problem if I also have heavy luggage to carry.

Another form of pollution that joggers and walkers are exposed to is the exhaust from vehicles. In the small town where I live, one popular area for jogging and walking is a pretty road along a small river and town park, but I have yet to discover a time of day when traffic is light enough for really healthful exercising. The rule of thumb for avoiding vehicle exhaust is to be at least fifty feet away from it, and this is often not possible. City walkers and joggers have an especially difficult time avoiding airborne pollution, and it is hard to know whether the risk/benefit ratio is ever in their favor.

6. *Viral infections.* The flu or any illness that causes airway inflammation creates a likely environment for an EIA reaction. It is usually wise to decrease your level of activity even with a slight cold. You probably won't feel like exercising when you are sick, but you might feel guilty about it and think you should push yourself.

7. *Hay fever and other allergies,* all of which create inflammation and highly reactive airways, will increase the possibility of EIA, but there are now so many new treatments for these conditions that their interruption of an exercise regime should be comparatively minor. Of course, if you are actively sneezing, with a stuffy head and runny nose, your level of activity should be somewhat reduced.

Managing EIA

Pursed-Lip and Diaphragmatic Breathing

In the old days, if people exercised and got out of breath, they huffed and puffed a bit until their breathing got back to normal. Now breathing techniques and breathing exercises are part of every athlete's routine, and even the coaches at health clubs and workout centers will show you how to breathe as you use the machines and do the various exercises. If you do not know about these techniques, you are not breathing as efficiently during exertion as you might, and you are also missing out on an excellent relaxation technique.

Pursed-lip and diaphragmatic breathing, of course, are not just for athletes; as we discussed in Chapter 17, they should be a standard part of every asthmatic's equipment and practiced regularly on a daily basis.

Premedication

When discussing an exercise program with your doctor or respiratory rehab nurse/therapist, be sure you understand about premedication; taking it at the time of your activities will be mostly your responsibility. If it doesn't seem to be working, do not hesitate to go back for further instruction or discussion.

Generally, premedication consists of using an inhaler about a half hour before you start exercising. If you have forgotten to do this and you start to have a problem, you can probably stop and use your inhaler then. Forgetting is sometimes a form of denial, unconsciously deliberate on your part, but it isn't smart.

If you want to try controlling EIA with nonpharmacological methods (without using drugs), find a doctor who understands this method. It will involve extensive training on your part in special breathing techniques, long warm-ups, limited exercise periods, and sometimes alternative methods such as hypnotism. A good compromise might be a combination of some of these techniques and medication. The better you can manage your asthma, the more you are likely to be able to reduce the amount and frequency of the medication you need.

Premedication is in addition to, not instead of, your maintenance use of your regular medication. Ask your doctor about it so that you aren't concerned, for instance, that you are overusing the inhaler.

Sympathomimetic (Adrenalin-like) inhalers, such as albuterol, metaproterenol, and terbutaline, are most generally used in the United States for premedication, but cromolyn sodium is preferred by some physicians and is sometimes even more effective. If you have both with you, remember that the cromolyn sodium is primarily for preventive use and is not effective when bronchospasm is already present. At that point only the albuterol (or some other bronchodilator) will relax your airway muscles.

Warm-up and Cool-down

Whatever exercise you do, start slowly and build up to a faster pace. When you stop, do it gradually. This is a good rule for everyone, but it is particularly important for asthmatics. The slow buildup may make a big difference in how your body, including your heart and lungs, handles the increased activity (and the need for increased oxygen), and it will also provide an opportunity for pursed-lip and diaphragmatic breathing if needed. The cool-down is especially important for your body's adjustment to a lower level of activity. When figuring duration, as in a twenty-minute aerobic stationary bike workout, do not include the warm-up and cool-down time in the twenty minutes.

Recreational Exercises

When you first start exercising, choose noncompetitive activities where there is no one else setting the pace. Walking and swimming are among the easiest. No matter how deconditioned you are, they are good for general conditioning, they can be done at any age, and the duration and rate of exertion are easily tailored to the individual.

Walking

In an age when exercise equipment has become increasingly complicated and sophisticated, walking stands alone as an activity that human beings come already fully equipped to do. By "shanks' mare" (on our own two legs) was the earliest way of getting from one place to another, and our increasing dependence on other methods has been responsible for much of the poor physical condition we find ourselves in today.

Walking feels good. Unlike so many "modern" exercises, it is gain *without* pain. Swimming comes close, but it will not flatten your stomach as walking will. Walking will also slim thighs and hips, tone up your muscles, and strengthen your heart and lungs.

If you walk a lot, a pair of walking shoes are a good investment. In cold or windy weather wear a neck gaiter, which not only keeps your neck warmer than a scarf but is much easier to pull up over your mouth and nose, providing warm air for breathing, and keeping out the wind.

If you haven't been doing much exercise, don't take too long a walk at first. There's a formula for the rate at which to increase distances or time spent walking (your rehab therapist may have a chart). The trick is to keep up with the level of your conditioning; in other words, as you become more fit you need to go farther or faster to continue improving. A walk to the corner may have been all you could do for the first week, but a mile may be your goal a few short weeks later. If you continue to exercise only at the level your body has already adjusted to, you will maintain the level of fitness you have reached but you won't go any higher. The aim is to reach maximum fitness, whatever that may mean for you.

Variations on Walking   Walking lends itself to many variations. First of all, unlike equipment-oriented exercise that must be done indoors, the setting can be a sandy beach, a woodland path, or a city street. It can be done any time of the day and in almost any weather. (When it is raining or stormy, many people like to walk in shopping malls.) And it can be done alone or with an agreeable companion.

Walking is not limited by the clock. A walk can last minutes or hours, depending on health, opportunity, and inclination. Your therapist may set certain limits, but once you are fairly fit, those limits are usually minimums and you can continue this pleasurable occupation as long as you wish.

The pace of walking is important for training purposes; your regimen will specify both the distance and the time in which it should be covered. But after you have met those requirements, you are free to take a stroll just to enjoy a particularly beautiful day or scenery, and even though you do it for pure pleasure, that will be additional exercise.

Once you loosen up and are walking comfortably at your pace for the day, swing your arms and get your upper body into the act. If your therapist agrees, you may even want to walk with weights. There are different kinds to choose from—weights you hold in each hand and those that go around your wrists. They are useful for other exercises, too, so get ones you like the feel and look of. I like the wrist ones: I can also put them on my ankles, so I get more use out of them.

Swimming (Noncompetitive)

The only drawback to swimming is that it requires a place to swim. If you live near a YMCA, chances are it has a pool and you can usually join for a modest fee. If you live near a lake or the beach, you can swim in the summer, but that can be a comparatively short period, and you are left at loose ends the rest of the year.

In some ways an indoor pool is better than the beach or an outdoor pool. Not only is it available year-round but the water is heated, and the humid air, which makes swimming such a desirable activity for asthmatics, is more pronounced. In outdoor swimming facilities the water is sometimes a little cold, which may bother your breathing. Also, if it is a windy day, you may get chilled coming out of the water or find the windblown sand or dust bothersome.

A possibly negative aspect of pool swimming (indoors and outdoors) is the chlorine-permeated air in the pool area. Some people with asthma are sensitive to it and cannot tolerate it for any length of time. Since I am not, I find the smell pleasant because I associate it with a sport I enjoy.

If you have an indoor pool available, try to choose a time when it is least crowded. Otherwise you may find yourself doing lap swimming in front of an aggressive swimmer who tailgates (or rather, heelgates) you in an effort to make you speed up. If this happens, do what a smart turnpike driver does in similar circumstances: slow down even more, and your heelgating speed demon will soon switch to another lane. Never react by pushing yourself beyond what you know is your maximum pace for that day.

When you first start swimming, the tendency may be to stop and rest at the end of every lap, or maybe even sooner. If you have to, that is all right in the beginning, but to get the most out of swimming as exercise, the goal should be lap swimming without interruption.

Once you are in the pool, there are many calisthenics and aerobic-type exercises that are designed for the water and are much easier to do than their land-based counterparts. Use them to warm up and cool down as well as for their own value. (Most therapists have copies of the exercises they recommend, or you can look up exercise books in the library.)

Some pools offer group pool aerobic classes that are excellent and fun. In addition to being healthful and less physically stressful than standard aerobics, they provide companionship, music, and variety. They are usually run by a physical therapist, and if you have an additional problem, like an aching back, the therapist will show you special water exercises to relieve it. Unlike other types of aerobic classes, these do not tend to set a fast, strenuous pace, and you do not need to know how to swim to take part in them.

By the way, if you do not know how to swim, it is never too late to learn. It is quite easy with professional instruction, and water is such a supportive medium that your muscles will not get stiff even if you exercise strenuously.

There are often bonuses to indoor swimming in the form of saunas, steam rooms, and tingling hot and cold showers. If you want to use a sauna or steam room, check with your physician to make sure it is recommended.

Indoor swimming plus sauna or steam room and after-activity showers need not dry out your hair; just rub on a little olive oil or hair conditioner before wetting down in the preswim shower.

Since most pools require a swim cap, the oil or conditioner will not get in the pool, and it will wash out easily in the after-swim shower, leaving your hair soft and shiny. To keep your skin from drying out, finish with overall use of a moisturizing lotion. (Asthma and allergies tend to be drying.)

If you take a swim, use the sauna and end up with a bit of this personal pampering; you will come out feeling as if you have spent a weekend at a spa. Think of it as a reward for doing such a good job of self-care of your asthma.

Dancing

If you like what used to be called ballroom dancing, you will be happy to learn that it is excellent exercise; it uses the same muscles as running or walking, depending on the speed with which it is performed. In addition, there are many modern exercise classes that utilize dance movements, such as "jazzercise," or jazz dancing, and as you probably know, most aerobic classes move to a loud, insistent musical beat that helps you keep the pace.

Folk dancing and Scottish dancing are more strenuous, but they are stop-and-go exercise, and no one will think anything of it if you sit out a reel or two. They also don't require that you come with a partner; you simply pair off for each dance, and everything is very informal. It's fun, inexpensive, and a good way to meet people. Check your local paper for a group near where you live, and go some evening to watch and see if it appeals to you.

Sports

Depending on the severity of your asthma, you may be able to manage your EIA so well that you can do anything you want, including sustained activities like competitive running or basketball. In the beginning, however, start out on a lower level with stop-and-go sports, which even though competitive do not require continuous activity. Golf, tennis, weight lifting, and even football fall into this category. If you have always wanted to try cross-country skiing but are a little dubious about being able to handle it, you could work out on a cross-country machine at a health club. It is very strenuous but, once you get the hang of it, has a pleasant rhythmic action and will condition all the muscles you need for the real thing. Needless to say, you will need the help of a trainer, both to learn how to use the machine and to monitor your pulse rate.

Calisthenics with Pursed-Lip and Diaphragmatic Breathing

Margaret Haggerty, coordinator of pulmonary rehabilitation at Norwalk Hospital, taught me a simple rule about pursed-lip breathing, "Just remember," she said, "exhale during exertion." I'm not always sure at what point an exercise is exertion, but I do know if I'm going up a flight of stairs, I inhale before I take the first step and exhale the rest of the way, unless it's a long flight of stairs, in which case I can stop and start again. I also learned not to hold my breath between breathing in and breathing out.

The following exercises are ones you can do at home, on arising (and before breakfast), for instance, to get set for the day ahead. If that is not a good time for you, feel free to set aside whatever time of day works best, provided it is before a meal or at least an hour and a half after.

To get the maximum benefit, exercise on a regular schedule, daily or every other day. The following exercises are only suggestions; your rehab therapist may suggest entirely different ones. (See also Chapter 17.)

1. *Relax Shoulders A.* When there is difficulty breathing, it's easy for shoulder and neck muscles to become tight. To loosen these muscles, consciously drop your shoulders with your hands down at your sides. In this position lower first one shoulder and then the other.

Next bring both shoulders up to your ears, as if shrugging; then slowly lower them to their normal position.

2. *Relax Shoulders B.* With hands at your sides put shoulders and arms back in a "parade ground" position (your chest will stick out). Then bring shoulders and arms forward; your hands will hang over your thighs, and your chest will flatten.

3. *Relax Shoulders C.* Stand up with your arms down at your sides. Roll your shoulders slowly and gently in circles (front, up, back).

4. *Relax Neck A.* With head straight and shoulders relaxed, turn your head left, then forward, then right, then front again. If your neck feels stiff, you might want to loosen it a bit before doing this exercise. (Incidentally, if it feels tight and stiff when you wake up, maybe you need a firmer pillow.)

Here is a good way to loosen your neck without straining the neck muscles: Lie on your back, head on a pillow, and relax head and shoulders as much as possible. Then place your left hand on your right temple and, using your hand but not your neck muscles, gently pull your head to the left. Repeat with the right hand on the left temple. Do not use any force, and keep all your head muscles completely relaxed so that you are moving your head entirely with your hand. Once your neck feels easier, you can get up and do exercise 4.

5. *Relax Neck B.* Standing or sitting in a straight chair, lower your head until your chin touches your chest. Raise your head, chin in, and lower it back as far as is comfortable. Do not strain. Straighten up and repeat.

6. *Tone Arm Muscles A.* With your hands down at your sides swing your arms alternately forward and back (one forward while the other is back), waist high in front and as far back as is comfortable. Continue this swinging movement as long as your therapist has indicated. (This is actually a Chinese meditation exercise called Li Chi and if done as a separate exercise can lead to a meditative state; ask your therapist if you want to try it for that purpose.)

7. *Tone Arm Muscles B.* Starting with both arms at your sides, swing them sideways, out and up, touching your fingertips over your head. Lower to sides and repeat. (You may recognize this as the arm movement in jumping jacks, but for this purpose do not jump.)

8. *Tone Arm Muscles C.* Lift your arms over your head, hands reaching for the ceiling. Make fists and bend your arms at the elbow, keeping your elbows close to your head and dropping your fists to your shoulders. Raise your fists to the ceiling again. This is an excellent exercise to do with wrist weights when you can do so comfortably.

9. *Flatten Stomach A.* Standing up, raise your leg off the floor, pointing your toe. Hold for a short count, then return. Do this with alternate legs. To strengthen inner and outer thigh muscles, repeat the exercise turning your ankle, first so your toe points outward. Do another series with your toe pointing inward. (If you put your hands on the muscles you are working on, you will feel them contract.)

10. *Flatten Stomach B.* Lie on your back with knees bent. Place your left hand on your left thigh and, lifting your leg slightly, press thigh against hand, resisting with your hand. Repeat with your right hand and right thigh. (To feel the stomach muscles contract, place your hand on the soft part of your stomach near the base of your thigh and below your abdomen.)

Turning Everyday Activities into Exercise

Once you start thinking exercise, you will find it is really a part of many things you do.

Walking up and down stairs. This is excellent exercise. One of the earliest American fitness specialists, a man named Bernard Macfadden, was a firm believer in stair climbing, and now that so many "old-fashioned" ideas have come back into vogue, the value of stair climbing is again recognized. Office workers are encouraged to walk up to their offices instead of taking the elevator, and in New York City climbing the inside stairs of the 102-story Empire State Building has been turned into an annual race.

If you have stairs in your home and have trouble climbing them, use your pursed-lip breathing. Inhale before you start and then walk up as many stairs as you can while exhaling. If you haven't reached the top, stop, inhale, and continue climbing while exhaling. You may be surprised to find how soon you are able to go up and down stairs without puffing, just by breathing this way. But it isn't a marathon, so don't push it, and stair climbing will get easier and easier.

Stretching. There are many opportunities for stretching: reaching for something on a high shelf, getting a medication that's rolled under the bed, scratching that hard-to-reach spot on your back—or just getting out of bed in the morning and reaching for the ceiling. Maximize every opportunity to increase stretch, and you'll gain flexibility and general muscle tone.

Do things the hard way. When you're feeling up to it, park at the far end of the parking lot and enjoy the short walk to and from your destination. Walk to the next bus stop instead of using the nearest one. Peel and eat a whole orange instead of pouring a glass of juice. Build in movement whenever you can. (Once you get to the point where you're cross-country skiing, you can go back to doing other things the easy way!)

Keep active. If you get a little stiff or feel a little cool because you've been sitting a while (watching TV, doing desk work, reading a newspaper, working at the computer), get up and spend ten minutes moving around briskly. Maybe bundle newspapers to recycle, file some reports, straighten out a room, fold the laundry, get a drink at the water cooler—it doesn't matter what you do (although it's a painless way to get small chores done); moving around gets your circulation going and will warm you up. If you absolutely can't think of a chore that needs doing, do a few exercises.

Part Five

Children with Asthma

19

The Asthmatic Child

A child with asthma has a lot in common with an asthmatic adult. He—or she—has many of the same symptoms from the same causes, takes the same medications, and from a surprisingly early age is able to understand, use, and manage inhalers on his own when away from home. But there are also many differences. A child is not a miniature adult, and no matter how knowledgeable you may be about adult asthma, there are special things you need to know in dealing with childhood asthma. Once you understand the differences, you can play a very important role in your child's health, his attitude toward his disease, and his future ability to cope with it. And you start out with an advantage that adults in a doctor-patient relationship don't always have: your child is dealing with someone whom he trusts and who he knows cares about him.

Choosing a Pediatrician

Choosing a doctor is never easy, but choosing a pediatrician for a child with asthma is especially difficult; not only do you want a good children's doctor but you need one who is knowledgeable about children's asthma and has kept up with the rapid strides that have been made recently in medications and treatment. Often asthma is not recognized if the doctor has not had considerable experience with it. Many asthmatics cough and wheeze their way through childhood only to discover as adults that their problem all along was asthma and was treatable.

The child cannot help, except indirectly, because he cannot evaluate the doctor and, when very young, cannot even articulate his discomfort or whether treatment is helping. A nine-month-old with asthma is basically helpless, and you have to take over the management that would be an older patient's own responsibility.

Fortunately, with a child of four it is a different story. He can understand a great deal about his problem and can be taught limited self-management, including the importance of taking medication as prescribed and using an inhaler correctly. You will still have to supervise the situation and keep a close eye on compliance, especially once school enters the picture.

Dealing with a teenager is different from any experiences that precede this stage. Teenagers tend to deny that they have anything wrong with them, and are notorious for not taking their medicine. They are not unique in this regard. Olympic medal winner Jackie Joyner-Kersee's husband described in a recent *New York Times Magazine* article how she often got herself into difficulties by neglecting her medication, and this is common with athletes and other mature adults as well as with children.

A good pulmonary pediatrician will help you deal with these various stages and advise you as to the best way to handle them.

Handling Yourself

A child with asthma creates an emotionally difficult situation to deal with. You should appear relaxed—as if you think there is no special problem and you know what to do even in the face of a severe attack. The reality is that you often feel frustrated because you cannot help as much as you would like; that, added to anxiety

Some Negative Facts About Childhood Asthma

- Asthma is one of the commonest childhood diseases. It is more common in children than in adults.

- If adolescents are included, it is estimated that nearly one third of the asthmatics in the United States are children; since the disease is often not diagnosed until adulthood, the incidence actually may be much higher.

- Asthma is the cause of 20 to 25 percent of school absences.

- It is estimated that childhood asthma is responsible for more than twelve million days spent in bed and more than twenty-five million days of restricted activity.

- Approximately 50 percent of childhood asthma begins before the age of three, but estimates are that about half to two thirds of all asthmatic children will outgrow it by adolescence. However, children with severe, early-onset asthma are less likely to outgrow it.

- Asthma is one of the leading causes of childhood hospital admissions.

Some Positive Facts About Childhood Asthma

- Asthma is reversible. With proper management most asthmatics can be symptom-free most, if not all, of the time.

- Having asthma doesn't mean not going out for sports. There are Olympic gold medal winners who have had asthma since childhood, and often the sports they excel in are the ones that most expose them to asthma triggers, such as horses and cold temperatures (see box "Olympic Medal Winners with Asthma," page 199).

- Exercise is good for children with asthma, even those with EIA (see Part Four).

- Many children "outgrow" asthma. One theory is that the airways get larger as the child grows, so there is more room for air to get through and less likelihood of mucus clogging.

- Asthma, even if severe, does not cause emphysema.

over the child's distress, may lead to behavior on your part that can actually make things worse. Since the child's attitude toward the disease will tend to mirror your own, anxiety, obvious worrying, and/or your own feeling of panic may create an atmosphere of tension and stress that can exacerbate the symptoms or make it difficult for the medication to be as effective as it might otherwise be.

The more you know about what to expect and what to do in various situations, what the purpose is of the various medications and how they should be used, and what the doctor's instructions mean—as well as what to do when you don't know what to do—the more relaxed you will be able to be. Be prepared; learn as much as you can about managing asthma. Make the most of the support system, both professional (doctors, school and other nurses, allergists) and personal (friends with asthmatic children, grandparents and other family members). Think in terms of setting a good example for the child by being cool and confident when symptoms occur. Since he will eventually be on his own, your ability to control his asthma will give him confidence that he can learn to do so too.

20

Helping the Asthmatic Child

It is estimated that two to three times as many boys as girls have asthma, but that statistic is reversed in adulthood, so if you have a boy with asthma, take comfort in the fact that he is more likely to outgrow it than he would be if he were a girl. One theory concerning the greater incidence of asthma in male children is that boys are generally more susceptible to lower respiratory tract infections than are girls.

The importance of these statistics to a parent is that they may make it easier to diagnose the problem in a boy. Asthma is notoriously difficult to diagnose in children because although the symptoms are the same as with adult asthma, there are a number of childhood illnesses, such as croup, bronchiolitis, and bronchitis, with similar symptoms.

Although asthma can manifest itself at any age, most asthmatics develop it before the age of five. Childhood asthma is most often, but not always, extrinsic or allergic asthma (although having extrinsic asthma does not preclude also having intrinsic asthma), so your pediatrician may wish to have a pediatric allergist as part of the team.

Once the diagnosis of asthma has been made, your pediatrician can describe how to recognize symptoms and what to look for. With so-called cough-variant asthma, for instance, the symptom may be coughing rather than the more familiar wheezing; however, the cough may also be a sign of asthmatic bronchitis, which is reversible but may be more serious. Both can be treated with asthma medications, but the child should be seen by a physician as soon as any persistent symptom is noticed.

An importance difference between child and adult asthma is that because of the child's smaller size (including smaller airways and less lung development) symptoms can develop dangerously quickly, and in the event of an episode treatment should be prompt.

Difficulty in breathing is usually very noticeable as the child labors to draw a breath, and a bronchodilator should always be handy so that there is no delay in reversing the bronchospasm and bringing relief.

Almost all the advice in this book for managing adult asthma is also applicable, with adjustments, to children. The difference is that children with asthma have special needs in addition to those of adults.

Eliminating Allergic Triggers

Most pediatricians and allergists will urge you to try to avoid episodes by keeping the child away from potential allergens as much as possible.

Obviously, a child with extrinsic asthma should not have pets, except perhaps for tropical fish. Puppies, kittens, and guinea pigs are all out of the question; even stuffed animals can cause problems if they are the furry type.

Since a child's room often doubles as a bedroom, study, and recreation area, it is especially important to forgo rugs and draperies (curtains that can be laundered frequently might be all right, but not those made of fabrics that have to be dry-cleaned, since dry-cleaning fluids are often triggers). Feather pillows should be discarded in favor of nonallergenic fillings, and sheets and blankets should be laundered frequently. Dust mites (in the parts of the country where they exist) can be a problem, and the room should be kept as dust-free as possible (difficult in a room with bedding), but never cleaned with the child in the room.

An allergist will usually have lists of dos and don'ts as guidance, and how far you take that advice will probably depend on the severity of the child's asthma.

Medications

Most (but not all) of the medications for adult asthma are used for children, but sometimes adaptations need to be made. For instance, a child under the age of four usually cannot learn to use an MDI inhaler, but spacing devices (Aerochamber, Inspirease), which eliminate the need for coordinating the release of the medication with inhaling it, can be a good solution. (Actually, many adults use spacers because they simply find them easier than trying to synchronize.) Quite young children can use nebulizers, and there are also syrups that are as easy to take as cough medicine.

Some children have difficulty swallowing oral medication, in which case the syrups and forms such as Theo-Dur Sprinkles can be used. In addition, there is often the option of mixing the medication with a spoonful of applesauce or something similar. (If you do this, try to get the entire dose in one spoonful so that it can be taken all at once. If it happens to be a time-release medication, for example, there would be a risk of the beads dissolving in a larger amount of the applesauce and releasing all the medication at one time—which could result in an overdose—or of the child refusing to finish the applesauce, thus not getting the full dose.) Any difficulty you have with getting the child to take medication, as well as any solution you invent to solve the problem, should be discussed with the pediatrician.

Incidentally, if you are the kind of parent who checks the *Physicians' Desk Reference* for medication information, do not be put off when it says a certain drug is "not approved for use for children under 12." This does not mean that the drug is not to be used for younger children but rather that the FDA has not had it tested for that age group. If a drug has FDA approval for one use, it generally means that doctors may use their judgment in using it in other ways. Medications are routinely used for younger children than the "under 12" note would seem to indicate.

Managing in General

With any chronic childhood disease, the family is likely to lean over backward in favoring the child. With asthma, it is especially important to proceed normally. Properly managed, asthma is generally quite controllable, and there is no reason why the child should be treated differently from any other child. You should resist the tendency to be overprotective and should allow normal activities, such as going out for sports and enjoying excursions with peer groups; normal, even strenuous, exercise is usually beneficial (when properly medicated and managed). In short, nothing should be done to undermine a child's feeling of confidence in his or her ability to control the disease.

You Are Not Alone

Since childhood asthma is so common, you need never feel alone. There are support groups you can join, and helpful newsletters are available (see Appendix 2 for names and addresses). For the child with severe, intractable asthma with which your physicians do not seem to be able to cope, there is always the option of the National Jewish Center for Immunology and Respiratory Medicine. It has done wonders with children of all ages, as well as with adults, and its achievements are world famous.

The Center is an impressive (but not forbidding) facility in Denver, Colorado, complete with swimming pool, an accredited school, and a special wing for teenagers, which looks more like a college dorm than a hospital. Because it is so highly specialized,

Managing Asthma at School

Teachers can be a big help, setting an example to the class and not drawing attention to the asthmatic child by being oversolicitous or fearful of having to cope with an asthmatic attack. Most children do not have severe attacks in school, and teachers and school nurses can easily learn the simple steps to take if one should occur. It is a matter of educating them beforehand so they feel capable of handling the situation.

It is unfortunate that some schools require asthma medications and inhalers to be left with the school nurse. The student then has to ask permission of the teacher to go to the school nurse even if all he or she needs is to take a couple of puffs on the inhaler. Not only does this draw unnecessary attention to a routine asthma treatment but also it is sure to cause the student to put off using the inhaler. Since it is important for prevention as well as maintenance, delay in using it is highly undesirable. Insistence on such an awkward procedure can also prevent the child from engaging in athletics (which may require pretreatment) and even, in some instances, lead to a full-blown attack (which could have been prevented simply by having an inhaler in the child's pocket, handy to use as needed).

Not all schools insist on this procedure, so it is obviously possible to allow the student control over his inhaler (and any other medication his physician and parents decide he is mature enough to use on his own). Parents might want to discuss this with school authorities if it is a problem.

all the latest equipment, therapies, and technology are available. It is research-oriented but so patient-friendly that it maintains a "Lung Line," accessed by an 800 phone number and staffed by registered nurses who will answer any question you have and, if by chance they don't know the answer—which seldom happens— will find out and call you back.

Doctors, nurses, respiratory therapists, and pulmonary rehabilitation therapists throughout the country have studied and trained here, and as far as I know, it is the only facility of its kind anywhere in the world.

The Center accepts both outpatients and inpatients, and the

staff works closely with your own physicians to coordinate the treatments they develop so that when the patient goes home, the care can be ongoing.

A book you might find helpful is *A Parent's Guide to Asthma*, written by Nancy Sander, the mother of an asthmatic child. It is full of down-to-earth advice and tips for everyday living rather than pharmacological and physiological information. Mrs. Sander is also head of an organization called Mothers of Asthmatics, Inc., which publishes a monthly newsletter (see Appendix 2 for information).

Part Six

Asthma Management in the 1990s

21

Looking Ahead, Looking Good

Great progress has been made in understanding and managing asthma in just the last ten or twelve years. Instead of a few combination drugs like Tedral, we now have a wide range of medications to work with. Instead of just oral steroids, invaluable but with undesirable side effects, we now also have inhaled steroids, with practically no side effects and great potential for long-range preventive results.

Research and development appears to be concentrating strongly in two areas, bronchodilators and anti-inflammatories. Not only are new drugs steadily coming on the market but the action and method of delivery of drugs already in use are being refined daily.

For example, Glaxo, taking to heart some patients' difficulty using metered-dose pressurized inhalers, has recently brought out Ventolin Rotacaps, with a Rotahaler that is breath-activated. And though the medication is in powder form, both the powder and the inhaler have been designed to eliminate some of the early problems with inhaled powder medications. People I have talked to who are already using Rotacaps report favorably on them. (One complaint I have heard is that it is expensive to have to buy the whole unit—both medication and inhaler—each time the medication is used up, whereas the availability of refills would reduce the cost considerably. Since refills are sold in Canada, it is possible they will one day be available in the United States.) The Rotahaler is very small and compact and slips easily into a pants pocket or handbag.

Another Ventolin (albuterol/salbutamol) breath-activated inhaler, also from Glaxo, which is not yet sold in the United States but is in Canada, Great Britain, and other countries, is the Ventodisk. (A steroid also comes in disk form as Beclodisks, for beclomethasone.) Both deliver the medication as dry powder in circular foil disks that fit into the inhaler. This disk type of inhaler is expected to be on the market in the United States in about a year.

Fisons, the manufacturers of cromolyn sodium (Intal), which some people found undesirable because the powder form made them cough, has reacted by creating a liquid form that can be inhaled just as other MDIs. And the number of forms in which other popular asthma drugs are now made shows that the manufacturers are really listening to user complaints and trying to respond with new designs and products.

Two new offerings expected out soon are Glaxo's Volmax (albuterol) and Warner-Lambert's Pro-Air (procaterol), and undoubtedly there are others in the works at other companies.

Improvements in bronchodilators are, of course, always good news, but anti-inflammatories, with their preventive function, may be the wave of the future. After all, if we could stop bronchospasm from occurring, we might not need bronchodilators. That is an unlikely scenario, but fewer episodes would certainly be welcome, and late-response asthma, which responds poorly to bronchodilators, requires the anti-inflammatories for real control.

Intense behind-the-scenes research is continuing on anti-inflammatories, but it seems to be directed more at arthritis and similar problems than at asthma.

For those with extrinsic (allergic) asthma who take antihistamines and have not been completely happy with Merrell Dow's Seldane (terfenadine), Janssen's Hismanal (astemizole) will be a competing nonsedating prescription product, as will Schering's Claritin (loratadine). From a consumer's standpoint, the downside of all these new prescription antihistamines is that their cost is on the high side, and OTC drugs, much less expensive, are likely to still have strong appeal in spite of their sedating effect.

Even those with good health insurance often do not have prescription drug coverage, and asthmatics—who tend to have multiple prescriptions that they take regularly—are particularly sensitive to high prices.

One of the most encouraging trends is the new approach to asthma that emphasizes prevention rather than after-the-fact treatment. This has grown out of new understanding of some of the physiological aspects of asthma, and its recognition now as an immune system disease. Since research in immunology is very active, asthma is bound to benefit both directly and indirectly. In addition, because a tendency to this type of disorder seems to run in families, gene researchers are also taking a look at it.

More interest is also being paid to nocturnal asthma; the National Jewish Center for Immunology and Respiratory Medicine recently completed an outstanding sleep center. Dr. Robert D. Ballard, who showed me through it, said, "We have been finding out some unexpected things about nocturnal asthma, and with this facility, we hope to be able to take it much further."

It is also good news that the myth of psychosomatic asthma, while not entirely dispelled among all members of the medical profession, is well on its way to wherever discarded theories go. You may still encounter doctors who think this way, but they are fewer and fewer.

And finally, there is a definite trend among asthmatics themselves to become knowledgeable about their disease. They are finding out that with good management really good health is possible for most of them. The future looks bright, with more and more people gaining control of their asthma and learning to experience wellness—not a neutral absence of illness but a positive state of well-being.

Appendix 1

Asthma Medications
Commonly Prescribed

New medications are constantly coming on the market, and many countries, such as Great Britain, are already successfully using some that have not yet been introduced into the United States. If you travel abroad, be sure you know the generic name of the medications you use—they may be sold under a different brand name in other countries.

Generic Name	Brand Name	How Used
Albuterol	Proventil Ventolin Rotahaler (Rotacaps) Diskhaler (Ventodisk)	inhaler, tablets, syrups
Bitolterol	Tornalate	inhaler

(*continued*)

Generic Name	Brand Name	How Used
Corticosteroid (beclomethasone diproprionate)	Beclovent Beconase Vanceril Vancenase	inhaler nasal spray inhaler nasal spray
Corticosteroid (flunisolide)	Aero-Bid	inhaler
Corticosteroid (triamcinolone acetonide)	Azmacort	inhaler
Cromolyn sodium	Intal	inhaler (spray)
Epinephrine (Adrenalin)	EpiPen	self-injection
Ipratropium bromide	Atrovent	inhaler
Isoproterenol	Medihaler-Iso Duo-Medihaler Isuprel Mistometer	inhaler
Metaproterenol sulfate	Alupent Metaprel	inhaler, tablets, syrup
Pirbuterol	Maxair	inhaler
Prednisone	Deltasone	tablets, syrup
Terbutaline sulfate	Brethaire Brethine Bricanyl	inhaler, tablet, injection
Theophylline	Slo-Bid Slo-Phyllin Theo-Dur	tablets, sprinkles

Appendix 2

Information Sources

Anyone looking for information about, or educational materials dealing with, asthma for themselves, their children, their relatives, or their friends, will find a host of organizations that devote their efforts to education and information through seminars, breathing clubs, free telephone consultations, and a wealth of materials in all media: books, brochures, video and audio cassettes, puzzles and games, and newsletters.

Some, such as the National Jewish Center for Immunology and Respiratory Medicine, through its Lung Line, and the American Lung Association, through its many local chapters, are especially accessible. But all are there to help; you have only to ask.

Here are some of the nationwide sources you can call on:

American Academy of Pediatrics

A teaching comic book, "Captain Wonderlung: Breathing Exercises for Asthmatic Children," is available in English, Spanish, and French. Single copies are free. Write the Academy at Box 927, 141 NW Point Boulevard, Elk Grove Village, IL 60007.

American College of Allergy and Immunology

This is a professional organization of physicians, teachers, and research workers in the field of allergy. For a list of publications, write: 911 Busse Highway, Park Ridge, IL 60068. The College also offers a card on sulfite sensitivity, and it has a toll-free physician referral number: 1-800-842-7777.

American Lung Association

(See Appendix 3 for local chapters in your state. Do not hesitate to phone the nearest branch for information or help.)

Founded in 1904 to fight tuberculosis, the ALA has 150 local and state Lung Associations throughout the United States. It is a very active and helpful organization interested in the control and prevention of lung disease. To this end it focuses on education, reaching out to the public by organizing and running local breathing clubs and offering lecture programs by area physicians, often cosponsored by local hospitals. It also makes available free literature on various aspects of asthma (and other lung diseases), and some of the local chapters have newsletters.

Additional available literature includes *Superstuff,* a kit for families with asthmatic children. It includes a newsmagazine for parents and educational activity material for children: games, puzzles, stories, posters, a record, stickers, and a personal notebook. Send $10 to Publications Department, ALA National Headquarters, 1740 Broadway, New York, NY 10019.

Asthma and Allergy Foundation of America

For information, speakers, and lecturers and a list of available literature, look in the white pages of your phone book, or write:

1717 Massachusetts Avenue NW, Suite 305, Washington, DC 20036.
Phone: (202) 265-0265.

Mothers of Asthmatics, Inc.

Founded by Nancy Sander, this helpful organization publishes a
newsletter as well as books for children with asthma and their
parents. For information about joining, or for a list of books and
materials, write Nancy Sander at the organization's headquarters,
10875 Main Street, Suite 210, Fairfax, VA 22030.

National Foundation for Asthma/Tucson
Medical Center

Inpatient care and an outpatient clinic for asthmatics are offered.
Booklets are also available, including "Asthma Fact and Fiction"
by Linda Alpert, with an illustrated list of triggers and information;
and "Dust 'n' Stuff" by Linda Alpert, instructions for dealing with
house dust and allergy-proofing the home, illustrated. Single copies of these publications are free. Write the Foundation at Tucson
Medical Center, P.O. Box 42195, Tucson, AZ 85733.

National Heart, Lung, and Blood
Institute

One of the federal National Institutes of Health, NHLBI offers free
booklets and information. Write NHLBI, National Asthma Education Program, 4733 Bethesda Avenue, Suite 530, Bethesda, MD
20814. Its National Asthma Information Center will answer questions if you phone (301) 951-3260.

National Jewish Center for Immunology and Respiratory Medicine

This is the world's leading and largest medical center devoted to the treatment of and research and education in chronic respiratory diseases and immunological disorders. It provides both hospital and outpatient services, and funds from contributions are available to help finance the cost of medical care for those who cannot pay all or part of the hospital charges. It is also an accredited Medicare and Medicaid hospital. The Center is deeply involved in research and in the investigation of new methods of treatment. It offers a number of free informational booklets and will answer lung disease questions if you call 1-800-222-LUNG.

For further information, write National Jewish Center for Immunology and Respiratory Medicine, 1400 Jackson Street, Denver, CO 80206.

Appendix 3

Associations Affiliated with the American Lung Association

ALA of Alabama
P.O. Box 55209
Birmingham, Alabama 35255
(205) 933-8821

ALA of Alaska
605 Barrow Street
Suite 2
Anchorage, Alaska 99501
(907) 276-5864

Arizona Lung Association
102 West McDowell Road
Phoenix, Arizona 85003-1213
(602) 258-7505

ALA of Arkansas
211 Natural Resources Road
Little Rock, Arkansas 72205
(501) 224-5864

ALA of California
424 Pendleton Way
Oakland, California 94621
(415) 638-5864

ALA of Colorado
1600 Race Street
Denver, Colorado 80206
(303) 388-4327

ALA of Connecticut
45 Ash Street
East Hartford, Connecticut 06108
(203) 289-5401

ALA of Delaware
1021 Gilpin Avenue
Suite 202
Wilmington, Delaware 19806
(302) 655-7258

ALA District of Columbia
475 H Street NW
Washington, D.C. 20001
(202) 682-5864

ALA of Florida
P.O. Box 8127
Jackson, Florida 32239
(904) 743-2933

ALA of Georgia
2452 Spring Road
Smyrna, Georgia 30080
(404) 434-5864

ALA of Hawaii
245 North Kukui Street
Honolulu, Hawaii 96817
(808) 537-5966

ALA of Idaho
1111 South Orchard
Suite 245
Boise, Idaho 83705
(208) 344-6567 or 345-5864

ALA of Illinois
P.O. Box 19239
Springfield, Illinois 62794
(217) 528-3441

ALA of Indiana
9410 Priority Way
West Drive
Indianapolis, Indiana 46240
(317) 872-9685

ALA of Iowa
1025 Ashworth Road
Suite 410
West Des Moines, Iowa 50265
(515) 224-0800

ALA of Kansas
P.O. Box 4426
Topeka, Kansas 66604
(913) 272-9290

ALA of Kentucky
P.O. Box 969
Louisville, Kentucky 40201
(502) 363-2652

ALA of Louisiana
333 St. Charles Avenue
Suite 500
New Orleans, Louisiana 70130
(504) 523-LUNG

ALA of Maine
128 Sewall Street
Augusta, Maine 04330
(207) 622-6394

ALA of Maryland
1840 York Road
Suites K–M
Timonium, Maryland 21093
(301) 560-2120

ALA of Massachusetts
803 Summer Street
South Boston, Massachusetts
    02127
(617) 269-9720

ALA of Michigan
403 Seymour Avenue
Lansing, Michigan 48933
(517) 484-5451

ALA of Minnesota
490 Concordia Avenue
St. Paul, Minnesota 55103
(612) 227-8014

Mississippi Lung Association
P.O. Box 9865
Jackson, Mississippi 39206
(601) 362-5453

ALA of Eastern Missouri
1118 Hampton Avenue
St. Louis, Missouri 63139
(314) 654-5505

ALA of Western Missouri
2007 Broadway
Kansas City, Missouri 64108
(816) 842-5242

ALA of Montana
825 Helena Avenue
Helena, Montana 59601
(406) 442-6556

ALA of Nebraska
8901 Indian Hills Drive
Suite 107
Omaha, Nebraska 68114
(402) 393-2222

ALA of Nevada
P.O. Box 7056
Reno, Nevada 89510
(702) 825-5864

ALA of New Hampshire
P.O. Box 1014
Manchester, New Hampshire
    03105
(603) 669-2411

ALA of New Jersey
1600 Route 22 East
Union, New Jersey 07083
(201) 687-9340

ALA of New Mexico
216 Truman NE
Albuquerque, New Mexico 87108
(505) 265-0732

ALA of New York State
8 Mountain View Avenue
Albany, New York 12205
(518) 459-4197

ALA of North Carolina
P.O. Box 27985
Raleigh, North Carolina 27611
(919) 832-8326

ALA of North Dakota
P.O. Box 5004
Bismarck, North Dakota 58502
(701) 223-5613

ALA of Ohio
P.O. Box 16677
Columbus, Ohio 43216
(614) 279-1700

ALA of Oklahoma
P.O. Box 53303
Oklahoma City, Oklahoma 73152
(405) 524-8471

ALA of Oregon
P.O. Box 115
Portland, Oregon 97207
(503) 224-5145

ALA of Pennsylvania
Olde Liberty Square
4807 Jonestown Road
Suite 251
Harrisburg, Pennsylvania 17109
(717) 540-8506

Asociación Puertorriqueña del
    Pulmón
GPO Box 3468
San Juan, Puerto Rico 00936
(809) 765-5664

Rhode Island Lung Association
10 Abbott Park Place
Providence, Rhode Island 02903
(401) 421-6487

ALA of South Carolina
1817 Gadsden Street
Columbia, South Carolina 29201
(803) 765-9066 or 779-5864

South Dakota Lung Association
208 East Thirteenth Street
Sioux Falls, South Dakota 57102
(605) 336-7222

ALA of Tennessee
P.O. Box 399
Nashville, Tennessee 37202
(615) 329-1151

ALA of Texas
3520 Executive Center Drive
Suite 100
Austin, Texas 78731
(512) 343-0502

ALA of Utah
1930 South 1100 East
Salt Lake City, Utah 84106
(801) 484-4456

Vermont Lung Association
30 Farrell Street
South Burlington, Vermont 05403
(802) 863-6817

ALA of Virginia
P.O. Box 7065
Richmond, Virginia 23221
(804) 355-3295

ALA of the Virgin Islands
P.O. Box 974
St. Thomas, Virgin Islands 00801
(809) 774-4624 or 776-5998

ALA of Washington
2625 Third Avenue
Seattle, Washington 98121
(206) 441-5100

ALA of West Virginia
P.O. Box 3980
Charleston, West Virginia 25339
(304) 342-6600

ALA of Wisconsin
1330 North 113th Street
Suite 190
Milwaukee, Wisconsin 53226
(414) 258-9100

ALA of Wyoming
P.O. Box 1128
Cheyenne, Wyoming 82003
(307) 638-63492

Appendix 4

Recreation Opportunities

Recreation is essential to a healthy lifestyle, but in the old days, having asthma was thought to mean that some activities were no longer possible. Today we know that activity and recreation are beneficial to an asthmatic and that it is usually possible for him or her live a normal, active life.

Cruises for asthmatic adults and camps for asthmatic children are two examples of the freedom that even someone with fairly severe asthma can enjoy.

Cruises

If you would love to take a cruise but hesitate because you don't know how you would manage if your asthma bothered you, you are in for a pleasant surprise. There are a number of cruises designed especially for people with just this problem.

As noted in Chapter 12, the trips are on regular cruise ships and most of the passengers are regular cruise passengers, but your group is escorted by a pulmonary physician and pulmonary clinical nurse specialist. In addition, oxygen and other respiratory equipment can be accommodated, and the cruise directors will assist with oxygen arrangements at airports and on flights. At sea you can participate in discussion sessions on relaxation techniques, breathing exercises, and other aspects of living well with asthma. You can also, of course, enjoy the usual cruise programs: the captain's cocktail party, late-night buffets, nightly entertainment, plus special social activities for your group. Both the doctor and the nurse are on call at all times, and all you have to do is relax and have a wonderful time.

An example of the kind of cruises available are the ones under the auspices of the Respiratory Health Association that go on the *Bermuda Queen,* with cruises from New York to Bermuda in the spring and from New Orleans to Mexico, Key West, Cozumel, and Cancún in the summer. For information on these cruises, call (201)-843-4111.

For other cruises, ask your hospital's pulmonary department or better breathing club which ones they sponsor or whether they know of others originating in your area. For instance, University Hospitals of Cleveland sponsors trips that begin from Fort Lauderdale, Florida, and cruise various Caribbean ports of call, including Jamaica and Grand Cayman.

Many people find that the confidence and know-how they gain from cruising makes it possible to travel to other places. Even if you need to take special equipment, the logistics can usually be worked out. And keep in mind that even though you can walk perfectly well, you should not hesitate to save your breath by using a wheelchair at airports to travel between your ground transportation and the plane.

Asthma Camps

The therapeutic value of exercise and physical activity for asthmatics of all ages has been clearly established; it is especially important that children with asthma be allowed, helped, and encouraged to exercise as much as they are able. Professional supervision under a respiratory nurse/therapist is the best way for you and your child to start.

Not only is exercise physically helpful in improving and managing asthma, it is also psychologically important in enabling children to join their peers in normal activity. The child who feels free to go out for team sports and become proficient in such skills as swimming, hiking, and similar activities that can be carried on into adulthood will gain confidence and a feeling of control, so that asthma will not be the focus of life but merely a minor problem to be dealt with.

If a child has mild asthma, a regular summer camp may be satisfactory, especially if the administration and staff are intelligent and generally knowledgeable about the usual childhood illnesses. If, however, a child has moderately or even seriously severe asthma, or is perhaps unusually apprehensive and sheltered, the camping experience is still available. The answer is asthma camps—camps specially tailored to the asthmatic child.

To locate a camp in your area, talk to your pediatrician and especially the respiratory nurse/therapist. There are asthma camps in almost every state, and many of them are run by the American Lung Association's local state chapters (see Appendix 3). Among the other organizations that sponsor summer camps are The Allergy Foundation, Asthma and Allergy Foundation of America, YMCA, University of Kentucky Medical Center, Asthmatic Children's Foundation of New York, Boy Scout Councils, and Children's Aid Societies.

The American Lung Association of Connecticut's asthma camps, for example, generally take children aged nine through thirteen and require physician approval. They offer twenty-four-hour on-site medical care, specially trained nurses, and respiratory therapists. Applications should be sent in early, since these excellent camps fill up quickly on a first-come, first-served basis.

In addition to enjoying a wide range of activities typical of a good camp experience, campers learn about asthma—early warning signs, triggers, and how to deal with an episode. Because they are part of a group of their peers, they do not feel awkward or uncomfortable learning about asthma but feel free to talk about it and discuss any fears or problems. They also see others actively participating in activities they may have thought were off limits for children with asthma, and thus they learn they can achieve success in many areas they assumed were closed to them forever.

Asthma camps can help children realize their full potential and can minimize the feeling of being helpless or in any way handicapped at a crucial period in their development. An asthma camp experience can truly change a child's life.

Most asthma camps are reasonably priced, and if needed, financial help may be available.

Although the greatest benefit of an asthma camp is to the child, do not minimize what the break will do for you and your whole family.

Appendix 5

Asthma Rehabilitation Centers and Programs

The number of asthma rehab centers and programs is increasing rapidly throughout the country. Those already in existence freely give their time and expertise to help train personnel from other areas who want to set up similar services. Many of these centers are associated with the pulmonary departments of teaching hospitals; some, such as Gaylord and Rusk, are separate rehab centers that work not only with asthma but with other types of illnesses and injuries. In every instance the goal is the same—to restore the highest possible quality of life to the individual, who can then maintain it through the education, support, physical therapy, and conditioning that is part of every program. There is generally a charge for some of these services; often insurance will cover all or most of the cost. Better Breathing clubs are free.

Since asthma is generally reversible and manageable, the potential for improved quality of life is high. Anyone who feels handicapped by this disease should make every effort to join one of these programs. If there is not one listed near you, get in touch with your local American Lung Association chapter; it may be able to tell you of one recently established in your area.

This list was compiled with the help of the American Lung Association.

Alaska

ALA of Alaska offers family asthma workshops in at least five communities every year. Most recently the communities included Anchorage, Fairbanks, Juneau, Kenai-Soldotna, Palmer-Wasilla, and Kodiak.

Colorado

National Jewish Center for Immunology and Respiratory Medicine
1400 Jackson Street
Denver, CO 80206
(303) 388-4461
National Lung Line: 1-800-222-LUNG

Connecticut

Bridgeport Hospital
267 Grant Street
Bridgeport, CT 06610-2875
(203) 384-3538
Evelyn Tkacs Cimmino, R.N.,
  R.R.T.

Danbury Hospital
24 Hospital Avenue
Danbury, CT 06810
(203) 797-7070
Techia Palmer, R.N., M.S.N.
Pulmonary Rehabilitation

Bristol Hospital
Brewster Road
Bristol, CT 06010
(203) 585-3000
Cynthia Buys, C.R.R.T.
Pulmonary Rehabilitation

Griffin Hospital
130 Division Street
Derby, CT 06418
(203) 928-6541
Sharon Garofino, R.R.T.
Pulmonary Rehabilitation

Greenwich Hospital
Greenwich, CT 06830
(203) 863-3170
Michael Marino, M.D.

Hartford Hospital
80 Seymour Street
Hartford, CT 06115
(203) 524-3637
Judy Randazzo, R.R.T.
Pulmonary Rehabilitation

St. Francis Hospital and Medical
  Center
114 Woodland Avenue
Hartford, CT 06010
(203) 548-4000
Jane Reardon, R.N., M.S.N.
Pulmonary Rehabilitation

Manchester Memorial Hospital
Hanes Street
Manchester, CT 06040
(203) 646-1222
Andree Guerette, R.R.T.
Pulmonary Rehabilitation

Meriden-Wallingford Hospital
181 Cook Avenue
Meriden, CT 06450
(203) 238-8220
Gail Brock, R.P.T.
Jan Vocola, R.R.T.

New Britain Memorial Hospital
2150 Corbin Avenue
New Britain, CT 06053
(203) 223-2761
Respiratory Therapy

St. Raphael Hospital
175 Sherman Avenue
New Haven, CT 06511
(203) 789-3995
Rebecca Stockdale-Woolley, R.N.,
  M.S.N.
Lung Life

Norwalk Hospital
Maple Street
Norwalk, 06856
(203) 852-2484
Margaret Haggerty, R.N., M.S.N.
Pulmonary Rehabilitation

Day Kimball Hospital
320 Humford Street
Putnam, CT 06260
(203) 928-6541
Maura Burke, R.R.T.
Pulmonary Rehabilitation

Gaylord Hospital
Box 400
Wallingford, CT 06492
(203) 269-3344
Margarita Rios, R.N., M.S.N.
Pulmonary Rehabilitation

St. Mary's Hospital
56 Franklin Street
Waterbury, CT 06720
(203) 574-6000
Betty Shreders, R.N.
Pulmonary Rehabilitation

Waterbury Hospital
64 Robbins Street
Waterbury, CT 06720
(203) 573-6000
Kathy Del Negro, R.R.T.
Pulmonary Rehabilitation

Windham Community Memorial
  Hospital
Mansfield Avenue
Willimantic, CT 06226
(203) 456-6788
Beth Wyatt, R.R.T.

Delaware

In addition to centers listed, the ALA cosponsors programs with local
hospitals.

Medical Center of Delaware
Washington Street
P.O. Box 1668
Wilmington, Delaware 19899
(302) 428-2988
Debbie Cebenka, R.N.

Milford Memorial Hospital
Clarke Avenue
Milford, Delaware 19863
(302) 422-3311, ext. 563
Sue McKinney, R.N., C.C.P.T.

Iowa

Pediatric Allergy/Pulmonary Department
University of Iowa
Iowa City, IA 52242

Kansas and Missouri

(Asthma and COPD pulmonary support groups are all free.)

Research Medical Center
2316 East Meyer Boulevard
Kansas City, MO 64132
(816) 276-4222
Pulmonary Services

St. Luke's Hospital of Kansas City
Helen F. Spencer Center for Edu-
  cation Board Room
Wornall Road at 44th
Kansas City, MO 64111
(816) 932-2737
Becky Martin, Pulmonary Reha-
  bilitation Program

Trinity Lutheran Hospital
Kansas City Regional Cancer
   Center Lobby
2940 Baltimore Avenue
Kansas City, MO 64108
(816) 751-2485
Melissa Matalone, Pulmonary Rehabilitation Program

Trinity Lutheran Hospital
Windjammers Club
3030 Baltimore Avenue
Kansas City, MO 64108
(816) 751-2485
Melissa Matalone, Pulmonary Rehabilitation Program

Mid-America Rehabilitation Hospital
5701 West 110th Street
Overland Park, KS 66211
(913) 491-2400
Rodney W. Hill, M.D., F.C.C.P.,
   Medical Director of Pulmonary
   Services

Kentucky

Our Lady Bellefonte Hospital
100 St. Christopher Drive
Ashland, KY 41101

HCA-Greenview Hospital
P.O. Box 370
Bowling Green, KY 42102

Medical Center
P.O. Box 90010
Bowling Green, KY 42101

Baptist Hospital East
4000 Kresge Way
Louisville, KY 40207

Frazer Rehab Center
220 Abraham Flexner Way
Louisville, KY 40202

Sts. Mary and Elizabeth Hospital
4400 Churchman Avenue
Louisville, KY 40215

Humana Hospital Southwest
9820 Third Street Road
Louisville, KY 40272

Humana Hospital Suburban
4001 Dutchman's Lane
Louisville, KY 40207

Lourdes Hospital
1530 Lone Oak Road
Paducah, KY 42001

Western Baptist Hospital
2501 Kentucky Avenue
Paducah, KY 42001

Michigan

Harper Hospital
3990 John R.
Detroit, MI 48201
(313) 745-1491

St. John Hospital and Medical
  Center
22101 Moross Road
Detroit, MI 48236
(313) 343-3769

Cardiovascular Health Associates
23133 Orchard Lake Road
Farmington, MI 48024
(313) 474-1614

Bon Secour Hospital
468 Cadieux
Grosse Pointe, MI 48230
(313) 343-1000

Cottage Hospital
159 Kercheval Street
Grosse Pointe Farms, MI 48236
(313) 884-8600, ext. 2161

Mt. Clemens General Hospital
1000 Harrington
Mt. Clemens, MI 48043
(313) 466-8078

St. Joseph Hospital—West
15885 19 Mile Road
Mt. Clemens, MI 48044
(313) 263-2484

Pontiac General Hospital
Seminole at West Huron
Pontiac, MI 48053
(313) 857-7324

St. Joseph Mercy Hospital
900 Woodward Avenue
Pontiac, MI 48053
(313) 858-3597

Crittenton Hospital
1101 West University Drive
Rochester, MI 48063
(313) 652-5644

William Beaumont Hospital
3601 West 13 Mile Road
Royal Oak, MI 48072
(313) 551-6038

Center for Asthma, Emphysema
  and Allergic Disorders
26206 West 12 Mile Road
Southfield, MI 48024
(313) 353-2270

Macomb Hospital Center
Pulmonary Clinic
11800 East 12 Mile Road
Warren, MI 48093
(313) 573-5277

Henry Ford Hospital
West Bloomfield Center
677 West Maple
West Bloomfield, MI 48033
(313) 876-1067

Missouri

The Asthma Center
Barnes West County Hospital
1040 North Mason
St. Louis, MO 63141
1-800-243-LUNG
Phillip Koren, M.D.

Montana

Deaconess Medical Center
2813 Ninth Avenue
Billings, MT 59101
(406) 657-4000
Jody Wingert

St. Vincent Hospital and Health
  Center
1233 North Thirtieth Street
P.O. Box 2505
Billings, MT 59101
(406) 657-7000
Paula Dowdle

Bozeman Deaconess Hospital
915 Highland Boulevard
Bozeman, MT 59715
(406) 585-1040
Karen Steiger

Deaconess Medical Center
1101 26th Street South
Great Falls, MT 59405
(406) 455-5240
Paul Kramer or Jennifer Grauptman

Health Promotion Center
310 Sunnyview Lane
Kalispell, MT 59901
(406) 752-5111
Deborah Wallen

St. Patrick Hospital
500 West Broadway
P.O. Box 4587
Missoula, MT 59806
(406) 543-7271, ext. 2074
Pam Gibbs or Randy Boehnke

North Valley Hospital
P.O. Box 68
Whitefish, MT 59937
(406) 862-2501 (Whitefish)
(406) 755-9206 (Kalispell)

Nevada

The ALA of Nevada offers an annual pulmonary rehabilitation program in Las Vegas.

St. Mary's Regional Medical Center
235 West Sixth Street
Reno, NV 89520
(702) 789-3270
St. Mary's Respiratory Continuing Care Service (RCCS)

Also: Nevada Respiratory Service, Inc., and Pulmonary Rehabilitation Department, Carson-Tahoe Hospital in Carson City.

New Jersey

These are actual rehabilitation programs, not basic educational programs, and do not include the ALANJ support groups. Call ALANJ for further information: (201) 687-9340.

Delaware Valley Lung Center
1155 Marlkress Road
Cherry Hill, NJ 08003
(609) 424-1777
John McCormick, Director

Elizabeth General Medical Center East
655 East Jersey Street
Elizabeth, NJ 07206
(201) 351-9000
Sue Yoon, R.N., Coordinator RESP Program

Breathing Center
95 Madison Avenue
Morristown, NJ 07960
(201) 539-5330
John Penek, M.D., Medical Director

Meadowlands Hospital
Cardiopulmonary Rehabilitation Center
P.O. Box 1580
Meadowlands Parkway
Secaucus, NJ 07096
(201) 392-3531
Doug Williams, Lifespan Director

New York

American Lung Association of New York State does not have a list of centers and relies on contact with respiratory and pulmonary therapy departments at hospitals. It is currently piloting an adult asthma exercise program and has started an asthma support club. Kenneth Scallion, director of programs for the state, suggests contacting ALANYS for Better Breathers and Easy Breathers clubs in local areas. Write him at 8 Mountain View Avenue, Albany, NY 12205, or call (518) 459-4197.

New York City Area

New York University Medical Center
Rusk Institute
560 First Avenue
New York, NY 10016
(212) 340-6117

Burke Rehabilitation Center
798 Mamaroneck Avenue
White Plains, NY 10605
(914) 948-0500

North Dakota

Heart and Lung Clinic
1006 East Main
Mandan, ND 58554

Oregon

(From their Better Breathers calendar; meetings are usually held at hospitals or clinics.)

Better Breathers—Baker
St. Elizabeth's Hospital
Information: (503) 523-1255

Better Breathers—Bend
St. Charles Medical Center
For information call: (503) 389-6358

Better Breathers—Brookings
Chetco Senior Center
Chetco Avenue
Information: Bill Lathrop, (503) 469-4932

Better Breathers—Coos Bay
Bay Area Hospital
Information: (503) 269-8069

Better Breathers—Eugene
Sacred Heart Hospital
Information: Ron Ballesteros, (503) 686-6858

Better Breathers—Grants Pass
Josephine County Health Department
Room 203
Information: (503) 474-5325

Better Breathers—Gresham
Viewpoint Room
Mt. Hood Medical Center
Information: Patty Brost, (503) 661-9287

Better Breathers—Hillsboro
Conference Room 2
Tuality Hospital
Information: Pat McClone, (503) 681-1111

Better Breathers—Klamath Falls
Klamath Room
Merle West Medical Center
Information: (503) 883-6227

Better Breathers—Medford
Smullin Center
Rogue Valley Medical Center
Information: Jan Young, (503) 770-5049

Better Breathers—Portland
Social Room
Providence Hospital Medical Center
Information: (503) 230-1111, ext. 5466

Better Breathers—Portland (veterans only)
V.A. Medical Center
ID132, First Floor
Information: Cathy Ponzoha, (503) 220-8262, ext. 6450

Better Breathers—Roseburg
Mercy Medical Center
Information: (503) 673-0611

Better Breathers—Salem
Community Education Center
Salem General Hospital
Information: (503) 370-5648

South Dakota

Rapid City Regional Hospital
353 Fairmont Boulevard
Rapid City, SD 57701
(605) 341-1000

McKennan Hospital
Cardiopulmonary Department
800 East 21st Street
Sioux Falls, SD 57117-5045
(605) 339-7677

Sioux Valley Hospital
1100 South Euclid
Sioux Falls, SD 57117-5039
(605) 333-6514

Texas

The ALA of Texas offers (a) Better Breathing Clubs for adults (often of retirement age) with asthma, emphysema, or COPD, (b) the Family Asthma Program for children and their parents, a six- to eight-week structured rehabilitation program, (c) the Asthma Support Group, a monthly meeting of parents with children, either alone or with the whole family, (d) asthma summer camps, and (e) school health programs.

To find out what is available in your area, contact:

Robin J. V. Anderson, R.N., B.S.N.
Program Administrator, Lung Health, ALA of Texas
P.O. Box 26460
Austin, TX 78755-0460
(512) 343-0502 or 1-800-252-LUNG

Utah

Cottonwood Hospital
5770 South 300 East
Murry, UT 84107
(801) 269-2701
Coral Kent

St. Marks Hospital
1200 East 3900 South
Salt Lake City, UT 84124

Utah Valley Hospital
1034 North 500 West
Provo, UT 84604
(801) 379-7165
Bart Brachen, M.D.

Washington

For further information and monthly newsletter:

Sara Swanson, Program Manager, King County/Northwest Region
American Lung Association of Washington
2625 Third Avenue
Seattle, WA 98121
(206) 441-5100 or toll-free: 1-800-732-9339

Auburn General Hospital
Auburn, WA 98002
Pulmonary Rehabilitation Program
(206) 833-7711, ext. 256

Providence Hospital
916 Pacific Avenue
Everett, WA 98201
Coordinator of Pulmonary Rehabilitation
Respiratory Care Services
(206) 258-7860 or 258-7387

Swedish Hospital Medical Center
747 Summit Avenue
Seattle, WA 98104
(206) 386-2187

Vancouver Lung Club
Vancouver Clinic
Vancouver, WA
Information: Renee Copen, R.N.,
    (206) 253-1255, ext. 1345

West Virginia

Plans are in the works for asthma camps and family asthma programs. For latest information, contact:

Shawn Harris Chillag, Program Director
ALA of West Virginia
415 Dickinson Street
Charleston, WV 25301-1771
(304) 342-6600

Breath Takers
c/o Florence Washington, Director of Pulmonary Rehabilitation
Wheeling Hospital
Wheeling Medical Park
Wheeling, WV 26003

Index